"I'm impressed. This is easily the most comprehensive and practical approach I've ever read on how to treat insomnia. I thought I had a pretty good handle on this topic, but was surprised to find large gaps in my knowledge, and quite a number of erroneous beliefs (don't tell anyone, please!). The authors expertly synthesize acceptance and commitment therapy (ACT) and cognitive behavioral therapy (CBT) (which is no easy feat) to offer effective treatment for a wide range of sleep difficulties across the whole spectrum of DSM disorders. So, if you want to help your clients to sleep better without drugs, you need this book."

—**Russ Harris**, author of *The Happiness Trap* and *ACT Made Simple*

"This fantastic toolkit is like getting to have two of the smartest, most empathic insomnia treatment experts in the world be your doctors. Clear instructions and flexible, doable steps transform the highest-quality treatment into a do-it-yourself plan that will make it possible to get a good night's sleep again."

—**Kelly Koerner, PhD**, Evidence-Based Practice Institute, Seattle, WA

"For those of us who lie awake at night wondering when sleep is going to arrive and what tomorrow will be like without it, *End the Insomnia Struggle* offers hope. In this well-written and accessible manual, Colleen Ehrnstrom and Alisha Brosse, two experienced clinical psychologists, take us through the reasons that people can't sleep, and the behavioral and cognitive strategies that help them overcome insomnia. Readers will appreciate the handouts for recording one's progress in the program and the many recommendations on how to troubleshoot one's sleep plan. The one-size-fits-all approach of many cognitive-behavioral manuals is replaced here with acceptance, mindfulness, and commitment strategies to help you individualize behavioral sleep tools. A must-read for people with insomnia and the clinicians who work with them."

—**David J. Miklowitz, PhD**, professor of psychiatry and behavioral sciences at the UCLA School of Medicine, Los Angeles, CA; and author of *The Bipolar Disorder Survival Guide*

"*End the Insomnia Struggle* is a wonderful and much-needed book. Ehrnstrom and Brosse not only provide clear descriptions of the core tools needed to help promote healthy sleep, they also pour into each page their wealth of expertise working with people struggling with insomnia. The result is that they are there with you, as the reader, every step of the way, guiding you clearly, firmly, and gently along the path to better sleep."

—**Sona Dimidjian, PhD**, associate professor in the department of psychology and neuroscience at the University of Colorado Boulder

"*End the Insomnia Struggle* is a must-have for anyone struggling to sleep well. Clinical science has validated a number of very effective strategies for insomnia, but unfortunately, these strategies are very challenging to put into action. The authors have put their combined forty-plus years of clinical experience into providing a comprehensive program in a very straightforward way that a motivated person can actually do on their own, or that counselors could readily use to guide their clients. The book is user friendly, and addresses all the possible excuses and roadblocks that might get a person off track. Their distinction between worry (future-oriented) and rumination (past-oriented) is particularly helpful. I have already made a list of family and friends to send this book to. Give it a try yourself!"

—**Linda W. Craighead, PhD**, professor of psychology and director of clinical training at Emory University, and author of *The Appetite Awareness Workbook*

End THE INSOMNIA STRUGGLE

A Step-by-Step Guide to Help You
Get to Sleep and Stay Asleep

COLLEEN EHRNSTROM, PhD, ABPP
ALISHA L. BROSSE, PhD

New Harbinger Publications, Inc.

Publisher's Note

Distributed in Canada by Raincoast Books

Copyright © 2016 by Colleen Ehrnstrom and Alisha L. Brosse
          New Harbinger Publications, Inc.
          5674 Shattuck Avenue
          Oakland, CA 94609
          www.newharbinger.com

Cover design by Amy Shoup

Interior design by Michele Waters-Kermes

Acquired by Catharine Meyers

Edited by Ken Knabb

Library of Congress Cataloging-in-Publication Data on file

Printed in the United States of America

24   23   22

10   9   8   7   6   5

Contents

PART 4: REVIEWING YOUR PROGRESS AND MAINTAINING YOUR GAINS

Introduction

*I*f you have trouble falling asleep or staying asleep, or you do not feel refreshed in the morning even after a full night's sleep, you are not alone. Insomnia is a large-scale problem, with one in three people experiencing insomnia in their lifetime, and about one in ten US adults reporting insomnia that is severe and chronic (National Institutes of Health, 2005).

You also are not alone in what insomnia is costing you. Are you exhausted during the day? Do you move more slowly and get less done? Do you have trouble with memory or concentration? Do you worry that others can see that something is wrong? Do you give up activities either because you are too tired or because you worry that the activity will make it hard to sleep? Perhaps you are more irritable than your normal, well-rested self. Maybe you have a lot of anticipatory stress and anxiety about how you will sleep tonight. Insomnia is not only about how you sleep at night. It is also about how you suffer during the day.

Nearly everyone struggles with sleep from time to time, but if poor sleep has become the new norm for you, you may have adopted some behaviors to try to cope (for example, staying in bed longer and longer). You also may be so worried about sleep that you are pre-occupied with thoughts about how you will sleep (*I have to sleep tonight, I just have to!*) or about the possible consequences of sleeping poorly (*Tomorrow is going to be awful!*). These behaviors and thoughts are perfectly natural responses to poor sleep—*and* they tend to make insomnia worse, interfering with your body's ability to naturally self-correct when sleep gets off track. Cognitive behavioral therapy for insomnia (CBT-I) addresses the thoughts (also called cognitions) and behaviors that influence sleep, helping people get out of their own way so their minds and bodies can remember how to sleep again.

Decades of research show that CBT-I works as well as sleep medications by the end of a six-session treatment program, and better than medications when people are interviewed a year after the program (Mitchell et al., 2012). Unfortunately, many communities do not have enough professionals trained to provide high-quality CBT-I, and some people cannot afford the cost of seeing a professional for six sessions. Fortunately, there are many books available to walk you through a standard CBT-I program. These books have been valuable resources for the millions of people who live with insomnia.

The Sweet Spot

So why another book on insomnia? About ten years ago we were approached by a psychiatrist who specializes in sleep medicine. He was desperate for people like us, clinical psychologists trained in cognitive behavioral therapy, to start providing CBT for insomnia. We dove in, excited to be able to offer a treatment that works so well for so many. For the most part, it was very gratifying work, because so many clients responded well and quickly to a brief CBT-I intervention.

However, we also met many people who claimed that they already had tried CBT-I—using a self-help book or very basic instructions from a doctor—without success. We started to see certain patterns, with two main groups of people for whom CBT-I did not seem to be working. The first group of people were those who did not really complete the program. Some became frustrated and gave up on CBT-I when they did not see quick results; others were too scared to fully implement the program, though they generally believed that they had done the treatment as prescribed. The second group of people were those who wanted the program to work so badly that they took it on like military boot camp—they tried very hard and followed all the rules very strictly. Despite all their best intentions and effort, their sleep did not improve, and their lives revolved around sleep, adding to their frustration.

We learned that there is a sweet spot. To successfully use CBT-I you need to:

- be strict enough with yourself that you are actually doing the treatment fully and it has the time it needs to work; *but*

- not so strict that your anxiety increases or that you do not allow yourself to adapt the treatment to your own unique situation and circumstances.

We teach people to achieve the sweet spot. We blend traditional CBT-I with parts of a treatment called acceptance and commitment therapy (ACT). The addition of ACT strategies has helped many of our clients become more *willing* to do CBT-I fully, and to stay *committed* through some initial discomfort, allowing them to benefit from the full power of CBT-I. We will be emphasizing willingness and commitment throughout this workbook. ACT also provides some additional tools for working with the thoughts that impact your sleep, such as mindfulness and cognitive defusion (chapter 12). Finally, ACT's focus on *acceptance* (chapter 3) has helped our clients decrease their struggle with sleep and with the daytime consequences of insomnia, changing their relationship with sleep.

You see, your relationship with sleep really does matter. If you try to control sleep, it may end up controlling you! Unfortunately, some people perceive CBT-I and other sleep strategies as more ammunition to control their sleep. We would like to suggest something different: think of all of our recommendations as strategies to *promote* (rather than control) sleep. The difference may seem subtle, but the result of this shift in perspective can be quite profound.

Who Can Benefit from This Book

This hybrid CBT-ACT program is specifically designed to help you with insomnia, which can be defined as difficulty falling or staying asleep, or nonrestorative sleep, with negative daytime consequences such as fatigue or difficulty concentrating. It is not likely to help you if you are sleep deprived simply because you do not have enough time to sleep.

If you can get plenty of good-quality sleep but only at a time that is out of sync with everyone else (for example, if your body can sleep 7 p.m. to 3 a.m., or 3 a.m. to 11 a.m.), you may have a circadian rhythm disturbance. Many people with circadian rhythm disturbances also have insomnia and can benefit from this entire workbook. However, only appendix A directly targets shifting your clock. We do not specifically address circadian rhythm issues related to jet lag and shift work.

Many people with disorders like sleep apnea, periodic limb movements, and restless legs syndrome also have insomnia, and can benefit from this book. However, these conditions need to be treated by a physician, and we encourage you to seek treatment before beginning this program (more on this in chapter 1).

If you have a medical condition like bipolar disorder or a seizure disorder, we strongly encourage you to use this book with the close guidance and supervision of a professional who is trained in CBT-I and has working knowledge of your medical condition. Some components of CBT-I will initially lead to less rest or sleep. This can make seizures and mood instability more likely in people who are vulnerable. With proper supervision, you can benefit from this program even with these vulnerabilities.

How to Use This Book

This book is not about what works for everyone. It is a book designed to help you figure out what will likely work for you, with your unique physiology, environment, and lifestyle. Unlike some CBT-I therapists, we do not believe that all people need every component of CBT-I, and we tailor the order of the different components or strategies based on our assessment of each patient.

To help you pick which parts of CBT-I are most suited to your sleep problems, in this book we will make extensive use of a sleep log and other assessments (chapter 1). Therefore, we strongly encourage you to read the next chapter and start to complete your sleep log before progressing to later chapters. Effective treatment begins with thorough assessment. Plus, CBT-I relies on ongoing information collection to help you guide the pace and direction of your program.

While you are collecting data with your sleep log, you can complete the rest of the assessments in chapter 1, learn about sleep and about what maintains insomnia over time in chapters 2 and 3, and start working on your relationship with sleep by reading chapter 4. Then, with information from your sleep diaries in hand, we will help you (in chapter 5) create an individualized treatment plan using the strategies outlined in chapters 6–12 that are most suited to *your* situation. You won't necessarily be reading all of these chapters. Instead, we will guide you to the chapters relevant to your individualized treatment program. Consistent with our goal of helping you individualize the treatment, with each part of the treatment program we will do a lot of "troubleshooting" to help you take into account your unique circumstances and potential roadblocks.

In chapter 13 we will ask you to reevaluate your sleep and will give you some suggestions for further steps if it is not where you would like it to be. In chapter 14 we will help you keep sleeping well by anticipating and protecting yourself against future sleep disruptors.

The last part of the book is devoted to topics that may or may not be relevant to you. We discuss circadian rhythm problems (appendix A) and insomnia related to menopause (appendix B) because we are so frequently faced with these issues when treating people with insomnia.

Your sleep will not improve just by reading this book. You cannot become proficient at any skill (knitting, woodworking, skiing, golf, swimming, cooking, and so on) just by reading about it. Rather, you have to have direct experience, and practice. Take your time working through this book. Answer the assessment questions we pose. Collect data for a couple of weeks. Work through the exercises in chapter 5 to develop an individualized program. Read thoroughly the chapters related to the strategies you select. Complete the worksheets that will help you personalize each strategy. (You can download the worksheets, listen to guided audio exercises, and access other related material at http://www.newharbinger.com/33438. If you are a clinician, you will find a bonus chapter on how to use this book with your clients.) Consider the possibility that the slower you go, the faster you will get to your goal.

We know how painful and costly insomnia can be. We are optimistic that, with our individualized approach that combines CBT-I and ACT, we can help you build and implement a treatment program that will enable you to sleep better and enjoy life more.

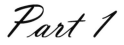

Part 1

LAYING A
FOUNDATION

Chapter 1

Taking a Look at Your Sleep

*I*f you have read other books on insomnia or talked with your doctor about your sleep problems, chances are you have been advised to do a number of things—limit caffeine and alcohol, have a wind-down routine before bed, use your bedroom only for sleep and sex, and so on. You may have found it challenging to navigate all the advice. (How much caffeine is okay? Should you really stop reading in bed even though it helps you get sleepy?) And since you really want to sleep well, you may have gotten focused on getting it "right."

Effectiveness as Your Compass

When we are asked a question ("Should I cut out my naps?" "When I wake up in the middle of the night, should I stay in bed or get up and do something?"), our most frequent answer is, "It depends." There is not a single right answer, nor a wrong way to do things. We can give you our best educated guess, based on what we understand about sleep physiology, and we will be doing that throughout the book. These recommendations will be helpful, on average. But you are not average. You are you. And you today, with your current health, life stresses, activities, and habits, are not exactly the same as you six months from now.

So when it comes to giving advice about your sleep, it is all about what works, not about rigid rules that apply to everyone. However, it is about what works in the long run, not just what works today. Things that give you short-term relief, such as a daytime nap, often come at the price of keeping insomnia around longer (much more about this in chapter 2).

We use the word "effective" to capture this idea of what works in the long run. You will notice that we use this word a lot in this book! We will help you use effectiveness as your compass to guide your treatment program.

But how will you know what truly works for you? Our mantra here is, *Collect the data!* And that is what this chapter is all about. You need data to help you choose the treatment elements best suited to your sleep problems, which will make this treatment work better, and more quickly, than a one-size-fits-all approach. Data also will help you monitor the impact of treatment, keep up your motivation, and guide the pace and direction of your program.

Sleep Log

A sleep log or sleep diary is the most important data collection tool for this treatment. It will help you recognize patterns in your sleep and track the impact of treatment. Because you will ideally collect data for ten to fourteen days before designing your treatment program in chapter 5, we want to encourage you to start now! In worksheet 1.1 we provide a sleep log that we have developed and tweaked over a number of years, as well as detailed instructions. We also provide an example of a completed sleep log. Take a look. A warning: the instructions are very detailed! We encourage you to take your time. You will get more benefit from your sleep log the more specific and accurate you are.

Once you have reviewed the log, instructions, and sample, return here for some additional guidance.

WORKSHEET 1.1: **Sleep Log**

Instructions:

1. In the upper left corner, fill in the date of the first day. This will help you keep your weeks in order.

2. Complete this log twice daily—at night (to record your daytime information) and again first thing in the morning (to record your nighttime information).

3. Fill in the days of the week that correspond to the hours of 6 p.m.–midnight, and to midnight–5 p.m.

4. Sleep Cycle: In this row, record information about when you are in bed, when you sleep, and when you wake up. Include both your nighttime sleep and daytime naps. Use this key:

   ↓   Time(s) you got into bed (at beginning of night, and if you leave and return to bed in middle of night).

   *   Time you turned the lights out (only mark if different from the time you got into bed).

   —   Time you believe you were asleep (use a squiggly line ~~~ to indicate light, fitful sleep).

   | Middle-of-the-night awakenings.

   ↑   Time(s) you got out of bed after lights out (including end of sleep period).

5. Medications: In this row, record all prescription and over-the-counter medications, including dose. You can create a key and use abbreviations (for example, m = melatonin; a5 = Ambien 5 mg).

6. C-A-N-E: In this row, record the time and amount of Caffeine, Alcohol, Nicotine, and Exercise. For caffeine and alcohol, list the number of drinks (for example, C2 means two cups of coffee or two Cokes; A3 means three beers in this hour). For nicotine, indicate number of cigarettes or amount of chew. For exercise, indicate number of minutes.

7. Hours Asleep: Record your best estimate of the total number of hours you were asleep *at night* (do not include daytime naps). Include fitful sleep (squiggly line).

8. Hours in Bed: Record your best estimate of the total number of hours you were in bed at night and *attempting to sleep*. For example, do not count time you spent reading in bed at the beginning of the night if this was simply part of your bedtime routine. Do count time spent reading if you were reading because you could not sleep and hoped to fall asleep while reading.

9. Fatigue: Rate the amount of fatigue you experienced on the day that corresponds to Midnight–5 p.m. 0 = No fatigue... 10 = Extreme fatigue.

10. Averages: At the end of the week, calculate and record your averages. (a) Add up your Hours Asleep and divide by the number of nights for which you have this data. Record your average. (b) Do the same for Hours in Bed. (c) Calculate and record your Sleep Efficiency (Average Hours Asleep divided by Average Hours in Bed, multiplied by 100).

Date: _____

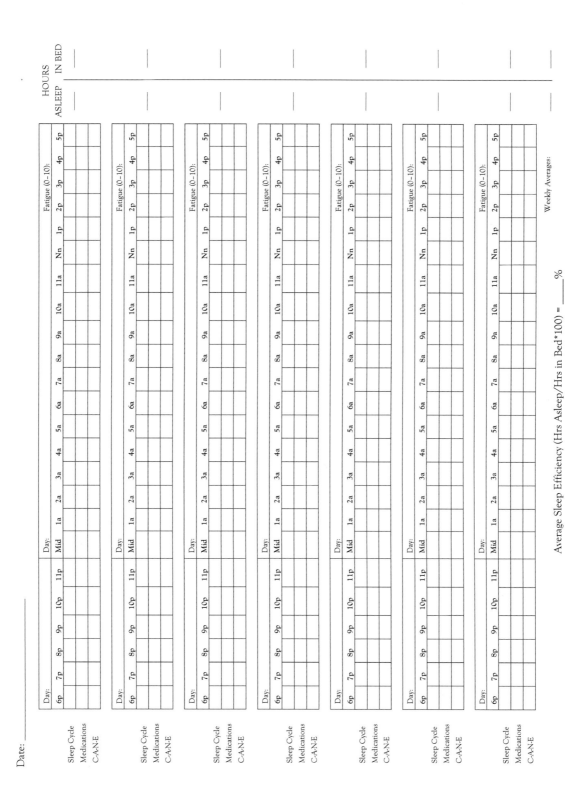

HOURS IN BED

HOURS ASLEEP

	Day:	6p	7p	8p	9p	10p	11p	Mid	1a	2a	3a	4a	5a	6a	7a	8a	9a	10a	11a	Nn	1p	2p	3p	4p	5p	Fatigue (0–10):
Sleep Cycle																										
Medications																										
C-A-N-E																										

Average Sleep Efficiency (Hrs Asleep/Hrs in Bed*100) = _____ %

Weekly Averages:

Sample

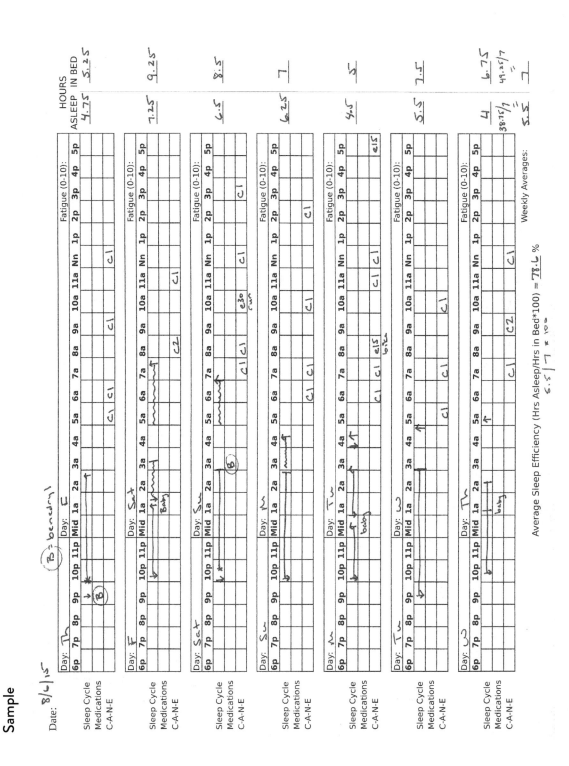

Common Questions (and Answers) or Roadblocks (and Possible Solutions)

"I do not want to look at the clock once I'm in bed. I'm afraid it will make me more anxious."

We agree that it is not useful to clock-watch. Fill in your sleep log as best you can, without getting caught up in having to be exactly right. For example, if you fall asleep around midnight and wake up at 3 a.m., and you know that you had two brief awakenings in between, put two vertical lines sometime between midnight and 3 a.m., even if you do not know precisely what time it was. Knowing that you woke twice is more important than knowing that you woke at 1:12 and 2:38!

Note, however, that people with insomnia tend to underestimate how much sleep they get. This means they overestimate how long it takes to fall asleep or for how long they are awake in the middle of the night. Therefore, you may decide to collect more accurate data.

If you do not want to look at the clock when you wake up too early, you can have a stopwatch at the ready. When you wake up, hit the start button. Then, when you get up for the day, you can see how much time has passed. If you get up at 7 a.m. and your stopwatch says two hours and fifteen minutes, then you know you woke up at 4:45 a.m. Or if you have multiple awakenings you want to record rather than just one, you can try what one of our clients did: he pressed the "memo" button on his smartphone any time he woke up; in the morning he was able to see the timestamp of all the memos he created.

A simpler option is to just glance at the clock. You may find that this is not nearly as anxiety provoking when you are doing it for the purpose of treatment, rather than wondering when the heck you are going to fall asleep!

Be flexible. If you are concerned about looking at the clock, try it both ways. Complete the log using your "best guess" for a few nights. Then complete it while tracking time for a night or two. Which do you think is more helpful? Does tracking time make you more anxious or alert? If so, are you willing to have a small uptick in your anxiety for a few nights? Or is the cost greater than the potential gain?

"I forgot."

Try to pair completing the sleep log with something else you do each and every morning and night. For example, if you use the bathroom morning and night, you can put on your bathroom mirror a sticker that reminds you to complete your sleep log. If you take medications or supplements at night and always start your day with coffee, you can put the sleep log or a reminder with your medications and near your coffee pot.

Leave your sleep log somewhere visible, such as on your bedside table. Have a pen or pencil with it. Some people like to have it on a clipboard, to make it easier to spot in a pile of clutter, and easier to write on.

You also can set a daily alarm on your watch or phone, or have a pop-up reminder on your computer. Pick the device you are most likely to see or hear first thing in the morning and later at night.

"I forgot for a few days. Should I go back and fill in the data that I missed?"

In general, we think that having no data is better than having inaccurate data. If you miss some days, fill in any information in which you are extremely confident. For example, if you use a pillbox and always take medications at the same time when your watch alarm beeps, you can look at your pill box and confidently fill in information about what medications you took when. Perhaps your exercise is in your calendar and you remember sticking to that schedule, and you can complete that. It may be more difficult to accurately recall how fatigued you were a couple of days ago, so you may want to leave that blank. In other words, do the best you can, but leave blank anything that requires guesswork. Our memories are quite fallible!

"Is it okay to complete the log once a day instead of twice?"

Most people find that if they try to complete the log only at night, they do not have as good a memory for their sleep the night before. So for most people we suggest completing the log soon after waking to record sleep the night before, and at night to record daytime fatigue and behaviors. If you find that in the morning you can easily remember all the information you need to record for the day and night before, then it is fine to complete it only in the morning.

"I don't have time."

After a couple of days of using the log it will probably take you one or two minutes at night and one or two minutes in the morning. Considering how important the sleep log is, and what your insomnia is already costing you, we hope you will agree that it is worth an investment of less than five minutes per day.

"I'm using a phone app or wearable fitness device that uses my movements to record my sleep pattern. Do I still need to complete this log?"

We strongly recommend that you complete a paper-and-pencil sleep log like the one we have included here. Different devices people use to record their sleep seem to come up with different results, and we do not know which devices or applications are most accurate. Also, some of the apps that our patients have used do not provide all of the data that you will need to guide your treatment program. Finally, using a log like the one we have provided may help you see patterns only obvious when you look at the data a week at a time, and with the sleep data right next to the data about the medications you took or other behaviors, such as alcohol and caffeine use.

"Should I track medications I take for things other than sleep?"

Yes! We encourage you to record all medications and supplements, whether prescription or over-the-counter. You may see that you are taking an activating medication (such as the antidepressant Wellbutrin [bupropion], or a decongestant such as pseudoephedrine) too late in the day. Or maybe a medication you take in the morning (such as a blood pressure medicine) makes you feel tired, so that you think you did not get adequate sleep, when really you did. You may want to consult with a physician or pharmacist to help you better understand the impact medications or supplements may be having on your sleep or fatigue.

"What should I include in my total Hours Asleep?"

Include all nighttime sleep. Include sleep that is fitful. Include sleep you got somewhere other than your bed. But do not include daytime naps. This means you are including all the time at night that is marked with a straight or squiggly line.

"Why should I count fitful sleep in my total hours of sleep? Won't it look like I'm getting more sleep than I am?"

You are right that it is not always clear whether fitful sleep should "count." We usually include it in the estimate of total sleep time because research shows that, on average, people with insomnia underestimate how much sleep they get. Also, as strange as this may sound, it is possible for you to be technically asleep even though part of your brain is alert and aware of passing time!

If you are concerned that counting fitful sleep will paint an inaccurate picture, then you can run the numbers both ways. Track your total sleep hours including fitful sleep, and your total hours of only more solid sleep. Then calculate two weekly averages—one for all sleep and one for more sound sleep—for both your total sleep time and your sleep efficiency. You will be able to decide over time which is the more useful or meaningful measure.

"Why should I track all of my time in bed, but only count in my total time in bed the hours that I am attempting to sleep?"

When we explain later in this book the theories behind stimulus control therapy and sleep restriction therapy, you will see that spending too much time awake in bed may be maintaining or worsening your insomnia. It is useful to see just how much time you are spending in bed. However, when calculating sleep efficiency, it is more useful to count in your total hours only the amount of time that you are attempting to sleep. You will be using your sleep efficiency data to help guide your behavioral treatment program.

"It is painful to see how poorly I'm sleeping. It stresses me out to look at the data."

Unfortunately, this work—whether it be the sleep log or the treatment program—may be uncomfortable or painful at times. We wish there was an easier, more comfortable, but just as effective way to help people with insomnia sleep better again. There is not. We hope it helps to know that this is likely to be short-term pain, with long-term gain.

"I just don't want to!"

It is your choice. You can choose to not track your sleep. You do not *have* to do anything we suggest. And not tracking will maintain the status quo. You are reading this book because you want something to be different in your life. It starts with *doing* some different things, even when you don't want to. The good news is that you probably have lots of experience doing things you don't want to do. Paying taxes comes to mind as an example!

Your mind can tell you, *Do not do it*, or *I don't want to*, and you can do it anyway. Try this exercise: say "I don't want to nod my head" three times, and on the second time, start to nod your head, even while saying that you don't want to. Silly, we know, but give it a try. What do you think: can you keep a sleep log even though you don't want to?

Are You Willing to Start the Sleep Log?

If your answer is yes, we encourage you to make some preparations to set yourself up for success. Download additional copies of the sleep log from http://www.newharbinger.com /33438. Decide where to put the log, and put a pen or pencil with it. Set up any reminders you think you need. Go ahead and get started! Then continue with the rest of the assessments in this chapter.

If you are not willing, carefully consider why. What are your specific concerns, fears, or obstacles? See if you can problem-solve or work through these. If you cannot (that is, you still are not willing), please skip to chapter 4 now. See if the discussion about acceptance and willingness increases your willingness to do the sleep log, even if just for a week. You do not have to commit to anything long term. You can collect some data about what it is like to collect the data!

If you still are not willing to keep a sleep log, you may benefit from using the skills in part 3 (Cognitive Strategies) to work with your beliefs about what it will be like or what it means to keep a sleep log.

You may be wondering if you can continue using this book *without* completing a sleep log, given all the emphasis we are putting on this. On the one hand, we do not want to lose you "just" because you are not willing to track your sleep. On the other hand, the data you can collect in the sleep log will help you choose the treatment components that are most likely to help *you*, rather than the average person with insomnia. We have found the sleep log to be a very useful tool in about 98% of the people we have been able to help. We want you to benefit, too!

Should You Have an Overnight Sleep Study?

As we said in the introduction, this book is intended to help people with insomnia. You may think you have insomnia but actually have a different sleep problem, such as sleep apnea, restless legs syndrome (RLS), or periodic limb movement disorder (PLMD). These conditions need to be diagnosed and treated by a medical doctor. If you have not had an overnight sleep study, or have not had one recently, review this section to help you decide whether to prioritize being evaluated by a doctor.

The first clue that someone may have sleep apnea, RLS, or PLMD is excessive daytime sleepiness. You are "sleepy" if you feel as if you could fall asleep. When sleepy, you may yawn, feel as if your eyes are heavy or droopy, or find your head nodding. This is different from being tired, exhausted, or fatigued. Many of our clients say they are exhausted but not sleepy. In fact, they yearn to feel sleepy!

To determine if you are sleepy during the day, ask yourself how likely you are to fall asleep in various situations, such as being a passenger in a car, listening to a lecture, reading a book, sitting in a dark theater, or resting at home. If you are very likely to fall asleep in a number of situations, we would say that you are sleepy.

It is natural for you to be sleepy during the day if you are not getting enough good-quality sleep at night. The question is whether your poor sleep and daytime sleepiness are caused by insomnia or by another condition masquerading as insomnia. Here are additional questions that we ask our clients to screen for sleep apnea, RLS, and PLMD. Take a moment to answer these questions for yourself.

Apnea

Do you snore regularly (more than three times a week)?	Yes	No
If yes, is your snoring loud enough to wake others?	Yes	No
Does your snoring wake you up?	Yes	No
Are you aware of waking up gasping for air?	Yes	No
Has a bed partner seen you stop breathing or gasp for air during your sleep?	Yes	No
Do you wake up multiple times a night?	Yes	No
Do you often wake up uncomfortably warm, even though the room temperature "should" be comfortable?	Yes	No
Are you overweight?	Yes	No
Has anyone in your biological family been diagnosed with sleep apnea?	Yes	No

We all have small pauses in our breathing while we sleep, but for most people these are very short and very infrequent. Someone with sleep apnea stops breathing for several seconds to several minutes, many times an hour. Most often people are not aware that they have stopped breathing, even if they wake up because of it. They may experience their sleep as restless, or say they have multiple awakenings throughout the night, or they may think they have slept solidly but feel unrefreshed in the morning. People with untreated sleep apnea usually feel very sleepy during the day.

If you are sleepy during the day and also answered yes to a number of the questions above, we strongly encourage you to consult with a doctor who is board certified in sleep medicine. He or she will ask a lot of the same questions and also will do a physical examination to determine if you should be evaluated for sleep apnea with an overnight sleep study. An overnight sleep study may be done in a sleep laboratory or in your own home using a portable device. If you do have sleep apnea, it is important to have it treated. Your doctor can help you find the best treatment for you (for example, a continuous positive airway pressure [CPAP] device, a dental device, or a positional device if you only have apnea when sleeping on your back). Many people with sleep apnea also have insomnia. Once your apnea is treated, if you are still having trouble with sleep, we hope you will return to this book.

Restless Legs Syndrome

When you are trying to relax or sleep, do you have an irresistible urge to move   Yes   No
your body?

When you do have an irresistible urge to move, does moving relieve discomfort   Yes   No
or odd sensations (such as pain, aching in the muscles, or a "crawling" feeling)?

Is the urge to move greatest at night, and least likely in the morning?   Yes   No

RLS is a condition in which you have an irresistible urge to move, especially when trying to relax or sleep. The urge tends to be greatest at night and most mild in the morning, and is most often experienced in the legs. Moving usually makes you less uncomfortable. If you answered yes to the above questions, ask your physician to evaluate you to rule out other causes of RLS symptoms, such as vitamin deficiencies. Some people get full relief by correcting an iron deficiency, for example. If you have RLS, a medication may give you some relief.

Periodic Limb Movements in Sleep

Are your covers a mess, or twisted around you, when you wake up?   Yes   No

Has a bed partner complained that you kick him or her while you are sleeping?   Yes   No

Periodic limb movements in sleep (PLMS) are repetitive, involuntary movements, usually in the lower extremities. You may recognize these movements as brief muscle twitches, jerking movements, or an upward flexing of the feet. However, most people do not even realize they are having them. In PLMD, the PLMS occur about every twenty to forty seconds. They can cause you to have difficulty staying asleep or may just compromise the quality of your sleep, which results in excessive daytime sleepiness. PLMD is diagnosed with an overnight sleep study. Some medications can cause the disorder, and the disorder can be treated with other medications.

If you are sleepy during the day and suspect that you may have sleep apnea, restless legs syndrome, or periodic limb movement disorder, please see a medical doctor for an evaluation. If, on the other hand, you are sleepy but answered no to the questions about these other conditions, your excessive daytime sleepiness may be caused by insomnia. It is reasonable to first try to treat your insomnia using this book. You can reconsider a sleep study if this treatment does not work for you, or if it helps you sleep longer but you still feel really sleepy during the day.

Do You Have a Circadian Rhythm Disorder?

In the next chapter you will learn about the relationship between your body clock ("circadian rhythm") and the external clock, and how our bodies generally are able to keep these two clocks aligned so that we sleep at night and are alert during the day. Even for people with body clocks aligned in the traditional way, there are individual differences: you may be a "night owl," a "morning lark," or something in between. An extreme version of being a night owl is called delayed sleep phase syndrome (DSPS). An extreme version of being a morning lark is called advanced sleep phase syndrome (ASPS). In both of these conditions, the body clock and external clock are misaligned: you can get enough sleep that is of good quality, but only at a time that is out of sync with the environment and cultural norms. For example, people with DSPS may sleep well from 3 a.m. until 11 a.m. if given the chance, but life demands may necessitate a 7 a.m. rise time. In an attempt to get enough sleep, they are likely to go to bed much earlier than 3 a.m., even though their body is not yet primed for sleep. It is not surprising, then, that they may have trouble falling asleep. This is often mistaken for onset insomnia (difficulty sleeping at the beginning of the night).

Similarly, people with ASPS may sleep well from 8 p.m. until 4 a.m., but life demands or social norms may cause them to stay up much later. Because their bodies are primed for awakening at 4 a.m., they may wake up at this time even though they went to bed later. This is often mistaken for "terminal insomnia" (waking too early and being unable to go back to sleep). Take a moment to think about your own body clock. To answer the questions below, consider your experience on vacations or when you have been able to set your own schedule, as well as what time of day you feel most alert.

If the world revolved around your schedule, such that you could sleep any time your body wanted to and you would not miss out on life, what time would your body most want to sleep? (Indicate a.m./p.m.)

Bedtime _____   Wake time _____

If you were able to keep this schedule every day without life interfering, do you think you would:

Get enough sleep?	Yes	No
Get good-quality sleep?	Yes	No
Feel rested upon awakening?	Yes	No
Be alert during your waking hours?	Yes	No

If your desired bedtime is before 9 p.m. or after 1 a.m., and you answered yes to the last four questions, you may have a circadian rhythm disorder. Some people who get properly diagnosed with one of these disorders decide to shift their lifestyle to accommodate their bodies' natural rhythm. Others attempt to shift their rhythm to be more in sync with the external clock and the people around them. We will address phase-shifting strategies in appendix A. Because many people with circadian rhythm problems also develop insomnia, you may benefit from working through the rest of this book, too.

What Is Insomnia Costing You?

To be diagnosed with insomnia, your disturbed sleep has to cost you something. We call these costs "negative daytime consequences." We are pretty confident that you have at least some negative consequences, because otherwise you would not be spending time reading this book! Still, we want you to pause and take stock. We will be asking you to take the same assessment at the end of this book, and knowing what has changed and what has stayed the same will help guide your next step. How does poor or unreliable sleep affect you during the day? How often? How much distress or impairment does this cause? Are you revolving your life around your sleep, so that you are living to sleep instead of sleeping to live?

ASSESSMENT 1.1: What Insomnia Is Costing Me

Think about how you feel and behave the day after a poor night's sleep. Also think about the overall, cumulative effect of your ongoing sleep problems. Now look at the list that follows of common daytime consequences of insomnia.

Circle the number of days in a typical week you experience each consequence *because of sleep disturbance*.

For any items you scored 1 or more, rate how much this affects you:

    0 = No big deal; I barely even noticed or thought about it until you asked.

    1 = Mild impact/somewhat distressing.

    2 = Moderate impact/quite distressing.

    3 = Significant impact/extremely distressing.

For example, if you are late to work three times a week, this may not be a problem at all because you have lots of flexibility and you do not mind shifting your work hours (0); or it may cause some personal frustration but no real problems at work or with your after-work plans (1); or it may cause problems with your boss/coworkers/employees/clients, or with other activities because you have to make up the time (2); or it may get you fired or make you lose business (3).

Because of insomnia I...	# Days in a Typical Week								Impact (0–3)
...am late to work, school, or other activities.	0	1	2	3	4	5	6	7	
...stay home from work or school, or cancel professional obligations.	0	1	2	3	4	5	6	7	
...perform below expectations or am less productive.	0	1	2	3	4	5	6	7	
...socialize less.	0	1	2	3	4	5	6	7	
...exercise less.	0	1	2	3	4	5	6	7	
...skip evening activities because I am too tired.	0	1	2	3	4	5	6	7	
...skip evening activities because I am worried they will disrupt my sleep.	0	1	2	3	4	5	6	7	
...have a harder time remembering things.	0	1	2	3	4	5	6	7	
...have a harder time focusing or concentrating.	0	1	2	3	4	5	6	7	
...am irritable with other people.	0	1	2	3	4	5	6	7	
...am more sad, tearful, or anxious.	0	1	2	3	4	5	6	7	
...worry about sleep during the day.	0	1	2	3	4	5	6	7	
...feel anxious about how I will sleep that night.	0	1	2	3	4	5	6	7	
...think about terrible things that may happen because of my insomnia (for example, impact on health, performance, relationships).	0	1	2	3	4	5	6	7	
...fall asleep at inopportune times (for example, during meetings or classes, or while watching movies).	0	1	2	3	4	5	6	7	
...am too tired to drive safely.	0	1	2	3	4	5	6	7	
...feel physically uncomfortable (for example, burning eyes or headaches).	0	1	2	3	4	5	6	7	

Your Next Step

In summary, if you have insomnia (trouble falling asleep, trouble staying asleep, or unrefreshing sleep) that is interfering with your functioning or quality of life, and you do not have signs of sleep apnea, RLS, PLMD, or a circadian rhythm disorder, continue to collect data with your sleep log while you work through the next two chapters. We will help you review and make sense of your sleep log data in chapter 5.

If you have signs of apnea, RLS, or PLMD, your next step is to get evaluated by a physician who is board certified in sleep medicine. If you think you have a circadian rhythm disorder, jump to appendix A. Even if you have another sleep disorder and are successfully treated, you may find that you also have insomnia that can be treated with the program in this book.

Chapter 2

How Sleep Works

We live in Colorado, a state with world-class skiing. We use the collective knowledge base about skiing to teach people about sleep. It sounds off-topic, but learning to ski—and specifically learning to ski off-trail and in the trees—can teach you a lot about sleep. When people are learning to ski this type of terrain, there is a natural concern about hitting a tree or other obstacles. As a result, novice skiers typically focus on the trees to avoid a collision. The journey down the mountain can be slow and anxiety-ridden.

More experienced skiers know that, to be successful, you need to focus on the space in between the trees. Your line of vision determines where your body goes. Your attention needs to shift from what you fear in that moment to where you want to be. Interestingly, even after skiers are told it would be best to shift focus, they still tend to look at the trees. It feels counterintuitive to not be acutely attentive to these large objects that would cause much pain if you were to collide with them. It is only over time and with repetition that skiers train their brains to shift their focus to the space in between the trees, allowing the trees to become part of the background. Concentrating on these open spaces allows for more freedom to create a continuous motion down the hill because you are now leading your body on the path of where you want to go, rather than avoiding where you do not want to go. It requires a willingness to trust in a process that does not immediately make sense to your mind. When this paradigm shift occurs, there is an "aha" moment, followed by an increase in confidence, ability, and enjoyment.

Sleep shares this paradigm. It is natural for people who are not sleeping well to become hyperfocused on what is going wrong, and to see danger or vulnerability around every curve. Yet this very vigilance can make sleep even harder, just like staring at the trees makes it more likely that you will run into one. Learning how to improve your sleep involves shifting your focus from fixing or avoiding your immediate sleep problems (the trees), to promoting and optimizing your healthy sleep (the open spaces). Concentrating on the components of healthy sleep will allow you more freedom to create a workable relationship with sleep, and a willingness to trust the process. When people make this shift in focus regarding their sleep, we typically get that same "aha" moment that leads to increased confidence and success (and, yes, even enjoyment) with sleep.

In this chapter we will discuss the "open spaces," or how sleep works when we are sleeping well. Remember: understanding what you are targeting (healthy sleep) will help you achieve it!

The Physiology of Sleep

Your sleep patterns are a result of a complex and impressive array of bodily and psychological processes. We do not review all of these moving parts in this book. Rather, we highlight what is most relevant for this sleep program. The two big players are your sleep drive and your internal body clock.

Your Sleep Drive

Your sleep drive (Borbely, 1982) is your body's personal tracker of your sleep. It is a drive because sleep is essential to survival: your body has an innate drive to get sleep in order to live. It tracks the amount of time you are awake and the amount of time you are asleep. When you are awake, your sleep drive goes up; as you sleep, the pressure valve is opened and your sleep drive goes down. When your sleep drive is high, your body will provide you with cues that it is important to go to sleep.

Your Internal Body Clock

Your internal body clock helps you navigate the cycles of day and night. This body clock is also known as your circadian rhythm (Halberg, 1969) and is responsible for the timing of your sleep. It is located inside your brain. Your body clock influences sleepiness and wakefulness by its impact on the endocrine system, the nervous system, and the body's core body temperature.

The endocrine system is responsible for hormones. The hormones that are most important for sleep include melatonin and cortisol. The nervous system is responsible for signaling to your brain how to respond to the environment, including when to react and when to relax. Your core body temperature is registered by your brain in tiny increments of tenths of a degree. Fluctuations significantly influence your energy and focus.

When everything is working well, day after day your body clock produces consistent fluctuations in cortisol and melatonin production, nervous system arousal, and core body temperature. You may experience this as predictable waves of energy and focus throughout the day. For example, you may notice feeling more alert and focused at midmorning and early evening, with a dip in energy in the late afternoon.

The body clock runs on a slightly longer cycle than our twenty-four-hour day. In fact, "circadian" literally translates to *about* a day." Remarkably, the human brain is capable of aligning these two clocks. This requires support from the environment. We know this from a famous experiment conducted in Europe in the mid-1960s (Wever, 1979). When people with healthy body clocks were put in a windowless basement for an extended period of time, their body clocks got confused. They no longer had a twenty-four-hour sleep-wake rhythm. It turns out that light exposure is a natural—and essential—regulator that keeps us on schedule. Nightfall is a trigger for us to sleep, and daybreak is a trigger for us to awaken.

There is variability in how robust the body clock is in handling environmental changes. Some people easily adjust to external clock changes, such as Daylight Savings Time or travel across time zones. People with robust clocks may feel fine with an irregular sleep or meal schedule. But others have greater difficulty adjusting to changes in the external clock, and may feel a lot more out of kilter when they do not have a regular routine.

A Well-Choreographed Dance

Understanding the interaction between the sleep drive and the body clock is essential to understanding how sleep works. It also is extraordinarily helpful in understanding your insomnia. The sleep drive and the internal body clock are two separate, independent biological processes, but they must work together in a complementary, synchronized fashion to support your wake and sleep patterns.

We can use the metaphor of meals and appetite to better understand this relationship. In many cultures the norm is to eat three meals a day, and the timing of these meals is typically in the morning, at midday, and in the evening. When your appetite is balanced, eating at the scheduled mealtime is something your body craves. It will provide you with cues, such as hunger pangs, at the time it expects food. However, if your appetite is out of sorts—perhaps because you ate a large meal or too many snacks—then eating at the scheduled mealtime will not be something your body craves. The more consistent you are with your mealtime schedule and the amount of food you eat at mealtime, the more balanced your appetites are. It is this synchronous process that allows you to know it is time to eat without looking at the clock. It also allows you to accurately predict how much food you need to prepare in order to be neither too hungry nor too full after your meal.

Your body clock and sleep drive work in a very similar manner to mealtime and appetite. In our culture the norm is to have a distinct wake cycle and a distinct sleep cycle. When your body clock and sleep drive are in sync, your body craves sleep at a consistent time. It will provide you with cues, such as sleepiness, at the time it expects sleep. If, for several months, you have kept a schedule of going to bed at 10 p.m. and rising at 6 a.m., your body will be primed to sleep during these hours. This is a synchronous process in that when you schedule the opportunity to sleep at roughly the same time each day, you have the necessary resources to do so. If your body clock or sleep drive are out of sorts—perhaps because you did not sleep well over the past few days or took a long nap earlier in the day—then sleeping at your regular time may become more challenging.

Figure 2.1 provides a visual depiction of the body clock and sleep drive, and how they interact with each other in a well-coordinated dance. This model is often called the "two-wave model," highlighting the fact that both the body clock and the sleep drive fluctuate in wavelike fashion.

Notice the lines crossing at the wake times and bedtimes. These intersections indicate a change in which another wave is dominant. The change sets in motion the wake or sleep pattern. At wake time, the body clock's signals for alertness are stronger than the drive for sleep, setting us up for the day. The body clock's alerting force remains the stronger drive throughout the day, allowing us to stay awake and focused, even as our sleep drive pressure mounts. At bedtime, the sleep drive becomes stronger than the alerting force of the body clock, setting us up for sleep. As we sleep, the sleep drive decreases. However, it remains stronger than the alerting force until morning. This allows us not only to fall asleep, but to stay asleep throughout the sleep cycle.

As you will see in the next chapter, this model helps explain how you can be extremely tired, yet be unable to sleep. You are tired because your sleep drive is high. You are unable to sleep well because your body clock is not primed for sleep. Your sleep drive and body clock are out of sync.

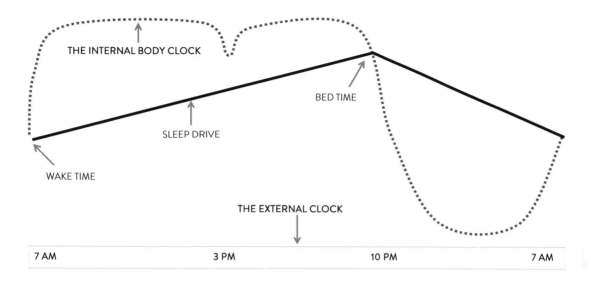

Figure 2.1. The 2-Wave Model of the Physiology of Sleep

How You Influence Your Sleep Physiology

We have already explained that the sleep drive is affected only by sleep: it gets stronger and stronger the longer you are awake, and steadily decreases as you sleep. We have also stated that there are individual differences in how robust our body clocks are, and how sensitive our body clocks are to the environmental cues of light and darkness. Maybe your mind has come to the conclusion that physiological aspects of sleep are "hardwired" and cannot be changed.

We have good news for you! Your behavior (what you do) and your thought processes (what, when, and where you think) also heavily influence your body clock and how it aligns with your sleep drive. Although you cannot force sleep, there is a lot you can do to promote it.

Behaviors that promote restorative sleep are designed to support your sleep drive and body clock. These behaviors support current restorative patterns, and encourage alterations in sleep patterns that have gotten dysregulated. They work at strengthening the body clock and the sleep drive, as well as the dance between the two.

In contrast to behaviors, there is not a prescribed set of sleep-promoting thoughts. It is not possible to force positive thoughts about sleep, or to simply will yourself to sleep. Check in with people who are sleeping well and you will hear them say that they do not think about sleep very much at all. Their general attitude reflects a sense of trust in the process of sleep. On the other hand, you, along with most people who are not sleeping well, probably think quite a bit about sleep. Or maybe you have a busy mind that keeps you up at night. Either way, these thoughts tend to be activating. This impacts the body clock in a way that can interfere with the "ideal" alignment of the sleep drive and body clock depicted in figure 2.1.

We want to help you support your body's natural capacity to sleep. We do this in chapters 6–9 by reviewing behavioral programs designed to promote sleep. In chapters 4 and 10–12, we will help you think more like confident sleepers do.

Your Next Step

Sleep is the product of complex relationships between the internal regulators in your brain, cues from the environment, and your behaviors and thoughts. These are ever-changing, dynamic relationships that have natural fluctuations. For example, your internal body clock changes over the course of your lifespan, with notable shifts in adolescence and late adulthood. You are exposed to more daylight in the summer and less in the winter. And life events are sure to interfere with "ideal" sleep-related behaviors and thought patterns. You will stay up late or wake up early to meet deadlines, tend to sick family members, spend time with family and friends, read wonderful books, or play enjoyable video games. These disruptions often are not avoidable. Even if they were, we would not want you to avoid life! We encourage you to check in with yourself to assess if you are sleeping to live, or living to sleep.

Fortunately, your body is designed to navigate these challenges. Sometimes you will return to restorative sleep right away. Other times, it may take a few days or weeks to restore your sleep-wake pattern. But rest assured, your body is well equipped to function in the real world.

If we are designed to manage these variations, why is it that we have such an epidemic of poor sleep in our culture? What is happening that your body is not able to resolve your sleep disturbance the way it is designed to? In the next chapter we will help you understand why your brain has not self-corrected, and you are instead stuck in an insomnia spiral.

Chapter 3

The Insomnia Spiral

*I*f we all have sleep disruptions from time to time, and our bodies are designed to navigate these challenges and self-correct, how is it that you are experiencing ongoing problems with insomnia? In this chapter we will answer this question by describing the 3P model of insomnia (Glovinsky & Spielman, 2006). We will then illustrate it with a case example. Finally, you will complete an exercise to make the model personal to you.

The 3P model, along with the two-wave model that you learned about in the last chapter, provides the rationale for all of the treatment recommendations we will be making in this book. We are sure you are eager to dive into treatment. Still, we encourage you not to skip this chapter! In our experience, this education will help you better understand the various treatment elements of this program. And this understanding can make all the difference in your willingness to do the treatment fully. Understanding the rationale also will allow you to make informed choices about when and how much to deviate from the recommended guidelines, and how to adapt the treatment in challenging circumstances.

As you work through this chapter, continue to complete your sleep log. You soon will use all the data you have been collecting!

How People Get Stuck

The 3P model of insomnia provides a framework for understanding how insomnia starts and how people get stuck. The three P's stand for *predisposing characteristics*, *precipitating events*, and *perpetuating factors* (namely attitudes and practices). As you read this section, refer to figure 3.1 for a visual depiction of the model.

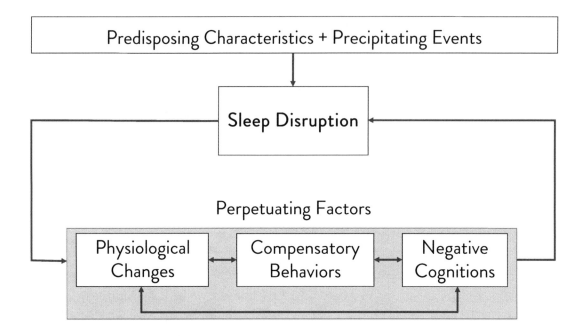

Figure 3.1. The 3P Model of Insomnia

The basic idea is that we all have characteristics that *predispose* us to develop a particular type of sleep problem. "Predispose" means to come before. Predisposing characteristics are present before you have a chronic sleep problem. They are risk factors. They may be traits that you were born with (such as being a "night owl" or a "high-energy" person) or that you acquired over time (such as an injury, or age). Predisposing characteristics do not automatically interfere with sleep, but they make it more likely that you will have sleep troubles. In less technical terms, we think of predisposing characteristics as "What You Had" leading up to your insomnia journey.

Precipitating events are whatever kicked off your sleep problems. These may be life events (such as becoming a parent or losing a job) or a biological process (such as menopause or an enlarged prostate). We like to think of precipitating events as "What Life Gave You."

"Precipitate" means to cause. In truth, precipitating events interact with your predisposing characteristics to create sleep disruption. For example, you may say something like: "I was always a bit of a night owl, but it was never really a problem until I took my first office job. Suddenly I had to be up by 7. I was exhausted by 11 p.m., but sleep just wouldn't come. I would lie in bed for hours." In this scenario, being a night owl predisposed you to—or put you at risk for—developing a sleep problem. Having to shift your schedule precipitated—or triggered—the insomnia. Here is another example: "I was always a light sleeper [*predisposing characteristic*], but I didn't have sleep problems until I had to sleep in a noisy dorm in college [*precipitating event*]. Now I have a nice, quiet home, but I still can't sleep."

As you have been reading, perhaps your mind quickly identified "What You Had" and "What Life Gave You." Maybe there is no way to change some or all of these things. Or maybe you do not want to change your triggers, such as working in a field with demanding hours, or having children. Or perhaps you have no idea why you developed insomnia, or why you developed it when you did.

Do not despair! You do not need to know, or be able to change, what caused your insomnia in order to treat it. Remember, our bodies are designed to self-correct—and sleep—even in the face of "What Life Gave You." Many people who are under tremendous physical or emotional stress have only a night or two of poor sleep. Then something in their brain says, *Sorry, pal, I need to sleep.* And they do. And many other people get back on track with sleep as soon as the trigger resolves, such as moving out of a noisy environment. So the real question is not why you experienced sleep disruption in the first place. The million-dollar question is, Why did you get stuck?

This brings us to the third "P," *perpetuating attitudes and practices*, or "What You Do." These are the thoughts you have and things you do in response to your insomnia. Your thoughts may be completely natural. Your actions may be completely sensible as you try to compensate for sleep loss. Natural. Sensible. Yet unhelpful, or even counterproductive. How can this be? This is because sleep is like skiing the trees. The interventions that help sleep get back on track are often counterintuitive. Choices we make to provide short-term relief in the moment (such as going back to bed, or taking naps) may work against what the body needs to return to its natural patterns (such as building a stronger sleep drive to get it back in sync with your body clock). This turns into a vicious spiral. We are trying to feel better and when our choices are not effective, over time we experience feelings such as anxiety, frustration, disappointment, and anger. These feelings then produce tension, which interferes with sleep. We continue to have poor sleep and we naturally have thoughts such as, *I will never sleep, Tomorrow is going to be awful*, and *Nothing is going to work*. This makes it even more likely that we will continue to choose behaviors that might provide some short-term relief but that, over time, confuse the body clock and deplete the sleep drive, maintaining our sleep problems. And the spiral continues.

A Case Example: How George Got Stuck

What George had. George is an active businessman who is always on the go. He runs an advertising agency and bikes five miles to and from work. He prides himself on his quick mind, working long hours, being creative, running a "tight ship," being liked and respected by his employees, and still having time and energy to spend with his wife and children. He generally sleeps well, and feels rested on seven hours of sleep each night. On occasion, he struggles to wind down from the day. On these nights, his mind is busy and his body is taut with energy as bedtime approaches. A little reading settles him down, and he falls asleep soon after he turns out the lights. We can describe George's predisposing characteristics as: high energy/intensity, high need for control, physiological hyperarousal, and an overactive mind (also known as "cognitive hyperarousal").

What life gave George. Five years into running his business, George and his wife decide to have a third child. They are very excited! However, their new baby has colic, and fusses much of the night. George finds that, even when it is his wife's turn to be up soothing the baby, he has trouble sleeping. Once he is awakened by the baby, he starts thinking about issues at work and how to solve them. It is 3 a.m., but his brain will not turn off. Although he has the opportunity to sleep approximately six hours per night, he is only averaging about five hours. He now has insomnia. His insomnia was triggered by caring for a newborn. Many parents in this situation would be *sleep deprived* because of the decreased opportunity to sleep, but would nevertheless sleep soundly when not up with the baby. George was vulnerable to this event triggering *insomnia*, and not just sleep deprivation, because of his overactive mind.

At this point, George's sleep problems are new. We can expect that they will resolve as soon as the baby starts sleeping better. It also is likely that George's sleep will get better even before his baby's sleep improves, as his brain's natural ability to adapt kicks in. George is confident that, like his other two children, this baby will learn to sleep, and then his own sleep patterns will be restored.

What George did. George was right about his baby's sleep improving. Six months later, she is sleeping much better. George is not. He wakes up most nights around 3 a.m., and his mind immediately starts thinking about work. Sometimes he remains in bed, tossing and turning, and finally getting some light, fitful sleep in the hour before the alarm sounds. Other nights he gets up and works at the computer.

Not surprisingly, George is really fatigued. His mind still moves quickly, but in a more frenetic kind of way. He feels less focused, and is a bit more forgetful. He tries to put on a bright face for his children, but his family can tell that he is less exuberant, and sometimes even a little irritable, with them.

George now has a chronic problem. He does what any of us would: he tries to fix it. George tries to manage his fatigue by sleeping in on weekends. He drives to work rather than biking. He gradually starts to drink more caffeine, hoping to get more energy and focus. He stops drinking alcohol, and has a regular wind-down period at bedtime. His disrupted sleep continues. He is confused about what is going on. He starts to feel anxious, and worries about the effects this sleep deprivation may be having on his business, and on his body.

Notice in figure 3.2 that What George Did impacted his sleep physiology. For example, his body clock is now primed to see 3 a.m. as a time to be awake and working. His body clock shifts when he drinks more caffeine, and when he conserves energy by reducing his exercise. Worrying about his insomnia further arouses him. What George Did also impacts his sleep drive. Sleeping in on the weekends depletes his sleep drive as he heads into Sunday night. He is so sleep deprived that his sleep drive still is higher than his alerting force at bedtime, so he falls asleep easily. However, because it starts at a lower place, his sleep drive is depleted enough by 3 a.m. that it cannot trump the message he is getting from his body clock to wake up and think about work. The body clock's alerting force spikes up above the sleep drive, and George awakens and cannot get back to sleep. He faces another Monday of sleepiness and difficulty focusing, and reaches for extra caffeine to get him through the day. And the cycle continues.

The very things George has been doing to help himself have now become a part of the problem. And the longer this pattern of thoughts, behaviors, and physiological changes persists, the more new data George's body is getting, and the more it will adapt to his new patterns, moving him further and further away from his more natural and workable sleep-wake pattern.

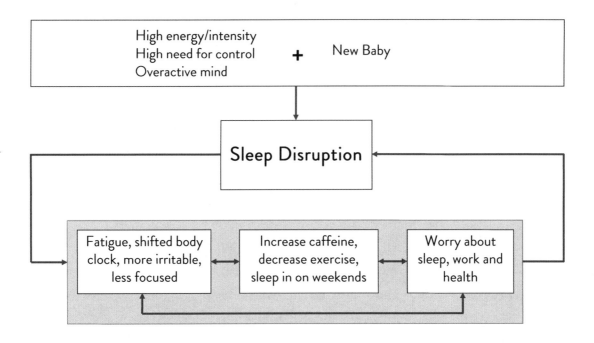

Figure 3.2. George's 3P Model of Insomnia

EXERCISE: How Did You Get Stuck?

Use worksheet 3.1 to take a close look at your own 3P's. What made you vulnerable (pre-disposed you) to developing insomnia? What, if anything, seemed to trigger (precipitate) your initial sleep problems? How are you responding to your unreliable sleep? Here are some typical things we hear. These are not exhaustive lists, so do not limit yourself to these examples when you complete the worksheet.

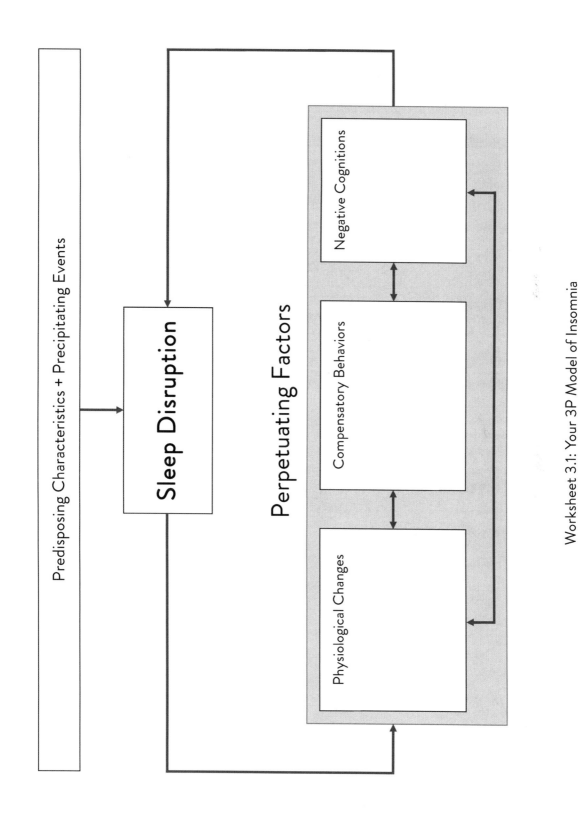

Predisposing Characteristics + Precipitating Events

Sleep Disruption

Perpetuating Factors

Negative Cognitions

Compensatory Behaviors

Physiological Changes

Worksheet 3.1: Your 3P Model of Insomnia

What I Had:

Poor sleeper all my life

"Light" sleeper

Worry or fret a lot

Chronic pain/discomfort

Depression

Anxiety

Hormonal fluctuations

"Type A" personality

High energy/intensity

High need for control

A body that tends to be ready for action (physiological hyperarousal)

A very active mind (cognitive hyperarousal)

What Life Gave Me:

Birth of a child

Death of a loved one

Increase in daily stress

Job promotion

Job loss

Moved

Financial hardship

Financial windfall

High conflict with someone

Health concerns/problems

Onset of menopause

Start or end of a relationship

What I Did to Handle Sleep Disruption:

Catch up on sleep by sleeping in on the weekends

Avoid scheduling morning activities for fear I won't feel up to them

Nap

Take sleeping medications

Watch the clock at night and get concerned as time passes

Avoid scheduling evening activities for fear they will interfere with sleep

Spend more time in bed

Watch television or play video games when I can't sleep.

Skip exercise the day after a poor night's sleep

Drink alcohol to sleep

Eat in middle of night

Cancel activities when I have not slept well

Increase caffeine/stimulants

A Balancing Act

Remember that "What You Had" consists of one or more risk factors, because these variables do not automatically interfere with the process of restorative sleep. Similarly, "What Life Gave You" may or may not impact your sleep. This variable, like the first, makes you more vulnerable to sleep problems. Similarly, no one thing that you did or thought in response to your sleep disruption is likely to be causing your sleep problems. It is all a delicate balancing act.

We use the equal-arms scale to illustrate this point. An equal-arms scale is the type of old-fashioned scale that has a beam anchored in the middle with one "arm" on each side of the beam. When you put objects on each arm, the arm with the heavier objects will tip down while the lighter side moves up.

On one side of our scale are things that promote or support restorative sleep. This includes aspects of your body clock and your sleep drive that are functioning well, and all the thoughts and behaviors that support and promote your sleep cycle. As long as this side of the scale is "heaviest," you will have restorative sleep. On the other side of the scale are all the variables that challenge restorative sleep. Medical and mental health issues, current environmental stressors, and the thoughts and behaviors that undermine or sabotage sleep are on this side of the scale. As long as this side of the scale is the heaviest, you will have sleep problems.

Stopping the Spiral

Throughout this chapter we have explored how your thoughts and behaviors interact with your physiology and sleep patterns. There is actually one more layer involved—time. The longer the spiral of thoughts, behaviors, and physiological changes persists, the more your body will pay attention. It is getting new data about your patterns of wake and sleep. So it does what bodies do. It adapts. Your body creates a new pattern based on the current cues from the body and the environment. It recalibrates and starts to identify these current trends as a new pattern. Sometimes this pattern has a known rhythm to it (such as napping during the day and awakening every night at 3 a.m.), and sometimes there is no obvious rhythm, so that you never know if this will be a "good night" or a "bad night." The common theme is that you no longer have predictable, restorative sleep.

Fortunately, we can change What We Do, and this is exactly what helps stop the spiral of chronic insomnia. CBT-I is focused on helping you identify the behaviors and thought patterns that were natural responses to your sleep problems but that have, inadvertently, "backfired" and become part of the problem. All of the interventions in CBT-I share the common goal of helping you reconnect and stay connected to the automatic and natural rhythms of your body. In chapter 5 we will build on the work you did in this chapter to help you choose the interventions best suited to stopping *your* spiral, so that you can return to a more restorative sleep pattern.

But first we must turn our attention to the topic of willingness. Remember our metaphor of skiing the trees? The end result of working on this skill is to become aware that you are in a forest that presents more risk than skiing on an open trail, and yet still be able to resist your urge to hyperfocus on the trees. Now you have a relationship with the entire mountain. This relationship is not built overnight, but over time, through consistent practice, skills, and willingness. Successful sleep is similar. Your relationship with sleep is lifelong, and you will do best when you are aware not just of this one night, this one urge, or this one feeling, but also are aware of how your choices today will impact your long-term sleep pattern. Although this paradigm shift is not part of classic CBT-I, we have found that it is essential to decreasing your struggle with sleep and supporting your willingness to do CBT-I.

Chapter 4

Willingness: The Opposite of Struggle

An art medium known as the autostereogram gained popularity in the United States in the early 1990s. A series of books and posters entitled "Magic Eye" was released. Autostereograms were three-dimensional pictures that "transformed" to a different picture when you shifted your perspective. There were instructions on how to achieve the proper viewing technique. You were encouraged to stand at a certain distance, soften your gaze, and patiently wait until the second image appeared. While some were able to find success quickly, a lot of people struggled. This struggle made it really challenging to soften and relax. Additionally, people reported that access to the hidden picture was often fleeting or inconsistent. These challenges could lead to a sense of defeat. Yet the pictures were a hit. The reward was worth the discomfort.

Managing your sleep problems can feel a lot like trying to figure out this Magic Eye art. Everybody has a recommendation or an opinion about what works. There is often a struggle with the prescribed guidelines. There is often this similar experience of inconsistent success. Yet despite the frustrations, we keep at it. We are compelled, again and again, to try to master sleep. This commitment to your sleep is likely contributing to your willingness to read this book right now.

You picked up this book because you are not sleeping the way you would like to sleep. You are reading this book so that you can design a program to promote more restorative sleep. Though CBT-I has been shown to be effective, it has two significant challenges. The first is that it requires you to be uncomfortable, both physically and emotionally. The second is that it requires you to trust in the process for a number of weeks before you see or feel any progress. This is going to be a struggle!

Willingness as a Tool for Sleep

We recommend a psychological tool that can support you when you find yourself struggling. It is a frame of mind that increases your ability to reach your goals. This is true whether you are trying to ski trees, see a magic picture, or improve your sleep. This tool is willingness. Willingness plays a key role in helping you achieve your unique balance of all the factors that keep your scale tipped in the direction of restorative sleep.

Willingness is often used interchangeably with the term "acceptance." Both terms imply the conscious choice to step back from our opinions and assumptions. This distance then allows us to view the world through a lens of objectivity. An example of this attitude would be: *I am willing to read this chapter right now,* or *I accept that I am reading this chapter right now.* It does not mean that you will like or dislike the chapter. It simply means that you are making a choice to engage in the process of reading it.

Willingness is not just a state of mind. It is also a state of action. You are open to reading this book. You are also, in this very moment, actually reading the book. We expect that you are also open to the content of this book. After all, you expect to learn something that will help you sleep. In chapter 2 we encouraged you to move from controlling your sleep to promoting your sleep. This can be a difficult shift, and willingness can help. Let's use the example of the toy known as the Chinese finger trap to illustrate how willingness can support this paradigm shift.

EXERCISE: The Chinese Finger Trap

The Chinese finger trap is a popular toy that is made out of woven paper or other stretchy material formed into a single tube. You place one of your fingers from each hand in each end of the tube. If we ask you to get out, or escape the finger trap, you will likely pull your two fingers away from each other, attempting to slip them out of the tube. When you do this, the woven paper tightens, forming a trap that prevents escape. You are "stuck" until you are willing to do what is counterintuitive: push farther into the tube. When you move your fingers toward each other, the tube loosens, giving your fingers more wiggle room. Even before there is escape, there is space. And in this space it becomes possible to leverage your fingers and remove them from the trap. Shifting your effort from pulling away to *leaning in* is what allows you to escape.

Willingness will help you to shift your perspective on how you manage your sleep. Willingness will help you recognize when your well-intentioned attempts to "fix it" backfire and end up feeding your insomnia struggle. Willingness teaches you to recognize this trap. Willingness helps you to end this spiral. It helps you to know when to lean in, rather than to struggle and fight.

Willingness creates not just a shift in perspective, but also a shift in action. This willingness involves choosing a different set of actions to promote your sleep. Specifically, we will encourage you to use willingness in two specific ways. The first is to be willing to make behavioral changes that are uncomfortable. The second is to be willing to not sleep.

Willingness to Make Changes That Are Uncomfortable

CBT-I relies heavily on behavioral change, and behavioral change is hard! Keeping a sleep log, restricting your time in bed, and skipping a nap are all examples of behaviors that are initially uncomfortable but can help you return to restorative sleep patterns. When you first read some of our suggestions you may react with something like *No way. I'm not doing it*. Or maybe you will consider doing it part way (for example, reducing your time in bed but not by as much as we suggest). Resistance like this is a natural part of behavioral change. However, you will need to be willing to endure the discomfort in the short term in order to achieve your goals in the long term. Your willingness to make room for your discomfort and frustration can significantly increase your ability to succeed with your program.

The Value of Emotional Discomfort

Have you ever noticed the double standard with judgments about emotional and physical discomfort? When we work on physical strength and fitness we are likely to experience discomfort, such as muscles aching or lungs burning. We consider whether this information signals if we are pushing too hard or not hard enough. Once we rule out any concerns such as overexertion or injury, we accept the discomfort. We label it as necessary to get stronger. We may even consider this discomfort a sign of growth. We have thoughts such as *I am really working hard now*, and *This is part of reaching my goals*.

Conversely, when we experience emotional discomfort (such as anxiety or frustration), we tend to immediately reject these experiences. We do not stop to consider if we are pushing too hard or not hard enough. We typically label all emotional discomfort as "bad" or "wrong." We assume the distress is a signal that something is wrong. This type of reaction feeds the spiral. It leads to activation and struggle and an instinct to pull back rather than lean in.

In our experience, willingness to experience both physical and emotional discomfort is a key factor in success with sleep programs. Practicing increased willingness will help you manage the moment-by-moment discomfort that naturally accompanies change and growth.

EXERCISE: Why Am I Willing to Be Uncomfortable?

When you notice this type of resistance, we encourage you to consider the long-term benefits that can be gained by being willing to have this short-term discomfort. You may want to think carefully about the following questions: *If I make this change, what will I have to give up? If I make this change, what might I have to experience? Am I willing to give up X? Am I willing to have Y? What do I hope to gain by giving up X or experiencing Y? How important are these gains I hope to achieve? Would it be worth it to give up X or to have Y if I knew I would make these gains?*

Remember George from chapter 2? One way he is coping with his insomnia is by increasing his caffeine intake. If he decides to reduce or stop using caffeine, he will be giving up the hope of increased energy and focus (X). He may be more tired and uncomfortable in the middle of his work day (Y). This does not sound so good! But then he considers what he stands to gain: making this change, as one part of his treatment program, may help him sleep better. And sleeping better will allow him to be the patient and focused parent and business owner he strives to be. Thinking of these potential gains, George is more willing to experience the discomfort of decreasing his caffeine use.

Here are some additional questions to ask yourself if, unlike George, you are still conflicted about making a particular change: *Can I be willing to be conflicted and still make this change? Can I try this, just to see what happens when I do something different? Am I willing to feel concern about being uncomfortable and engage in the program anyway?*

Willingness to Not Sleep

What? We're writing a book on treating your insomnia, and we're asking you to be willing to not sleep? That's right. Because that is the frustrating paradox: sleeping is one of the few things that becomes more difficult the harder you try. Sleep experts refer to this as "sleep effort" and have shown that there is such a thing as too much effort (Espie et al., 2006). Studies have found that when people consciously try to work harder at sleep, it invariably has the opposite effect (Ansfield, Wegner & Bowser, 1996). Therefore, we will ask you to be willing to shift your effort away from trying to sleep and toward behaviors and thoughts that will promote restorative sleep. The most optimal time to put forth effort around your sleep is during the day. We provide many tools and techniques for addressing your sleep needs, and though some of them require you to behave in certain ways during your sleep time, most of your effort regarding sleep is done during your wake time. This means that you will need to teach your mind to notice when and where the effort related to sleep works, and when and where it does not work.

EXERCISE: Tug-of-War

Let's try another willingness exercise. Grab something that could be used in a mock game of tug of war, like a piece of rope, a belt, or a dish towel. If you are around someone else, ask if that person would be willing to participate by playing the "Insomnia Monster"; otherwise, do your best as we walk you through this exercise to imagine someone on the other end of the "rope." Grab one end of the rope and have the Insomnia Monster grab the other end. Imagine that there is a big pit between the two of you, and you really do not want to be pulled into the pit. This pit represents all that you hate and fear about your insomnia. You will naturally feel some urgency to avoid this pit and will work as hard as you can to tug on that rope and avoid being pulled into the pit. You may even be hoping to pull the Monster into the pit! However, you are up against the Insomnia Monster—a creature with great power and strength. The harder you pull, the harder the Monster pulls. What do you do?

Most of us keep trying harder. We plant our feet and pull with all of our might, with our eyes fixed on the Monster. All of our resources go into our effort to not get pulled in. It is hard to imagine doing anything else. Yet there is another option. Do not play the game anymore. You can put down the rope. Are you willing to try this? If so, let go and see what happens. Notice what happens in your body and mind as you try this alternative approach. Notice that when you put down the rope, you no longer have to fear being pulled into the pit. Notice how your body can now relax. Of course, the Insomnia Monster cannot get pulled into the pit either; it is still there. But you now have your strength and energy to focus on something else.

Are you willing to drop the rope? Are you willing to practice reducing your sleep effort at night? Can you surrender to whatever this night brings?

Acceptance Is Not Resignation

When we ask you to be willing to not sleep, we want to be clear that we are not asking you to give up on your hopes and expectations regarding getting more consistent, good-quality sleep. Willingness and acceptance are about what is happening right here, right now. We are asking you to be willing to have whatever this one night brings. We are not suggesting that you resign yourself to a lifetime of sleeplessness. With resignation, you give up trying altogether. You do not even try to create or maintain healthy sleep habits, or to do a behavioral treatment program. We would not be writing this book if we thought you had to accept insomnia into your life forever! Paradoxically, being willing to not sleep (or not sleep well) on any given night allows you to relax into that night, to surrender, to decrease your sleep effort, and therefore your physiological arousal—making sleep *more* likely. Just like the finger traps; leaning into the space where you really do not want to be creates some wiggle room and allows something else to happen.

EXERCISE: Imagining Willingness

Imagine yourself in front of an autostereogram trying to see both pictures. Imagine yourself getting frustrated and responding by trying even harder to see both pictures. Now imagine asking yourself to be willing to accept that you may, or may not, see the hidden picture. Also imagine yourself continuing to stand in front of the picture, allowing for the opportunity to try and see what is right in front of you.

Now imagine yourself at the top of a mountain, preparing to ski a challenging tree run that pushes you to your limits. Notice yourself trying hard to manage your anxiety and fears. Now imagine yourself being willing to have those thoughts and feelings. Imagine yourself skiing down the mountain, allowing for the opportunity for an enjoyable experience.

Now imagine yourself preparing for bed and having thoughts and feelings regarding your upcoming sleep. Notice yourself trying to sleep and also notice your concerns and anxious thoughts about not being able to sleep. Now imagine getting into bed and being willing to have whatever thoughts, feelings, sensations, and experiences show up, allowing for the opportunity to build a healthy and sustainable relationship with sleep.

These shifts are not easy to make, even in our imagination! It requires time and practice to create this more willing and more effective stance. When you feel stuck regarding your sleep patterns, especially at night when you are trying to sleep, it is very natural to put in more effort, and try harder, and struggle. Can you lean into your experience instead? Can you give yourself more space, and be willing to have whatever this night brings?

Recognize How You Struggle with Sleep

In what ways do you pick up the tug-of-war rope? Think of situations where you feel locked in battle with your sleep problems. What thoughts do you have? What behaviors do you engage in? Do you toss and turn in bed? Do you give up on sleep by getting up and getting active during the night? Do you make choices during the day and night that you later regret (such as increasing caffeine, skipping exercise, or taking naps)?

Your Willingness Plan

While you are working through the next chapter, we would like you to practice "dropping the rope" and "leaning in." That is, if you catch yourself thinking apprehensively about whether or how you will sleep tonight, notice this struggle and put the rope down, or lean into the discomfort of not knowing. See if you can approach your bed with the willingness to experience whatever this night brings. You can do this same practice if you are lying in bed awake.

We have produced guided audio of a willingness exercise, which you can access at http://www.newharbinger.com/33438.

In the next chapter we will help you build your individualized treatment program. We hope that you will be willing to work a behavioral program and learn and practice cognitive strategies. By "working a program" we mean fully engaging with it. Throughout this book we will encourage you to keep checking in about your level of willingness. If willingness is low, you may want to reread this chapter. If you need additional support in increasing willingness, we think you will find the skills of mindfulness and cognitive defusion (chapter 12) especially helpful.

Chapter 5

Create Your Own Individualized Treatment Plan

*Y*ou may remember from the introduction that cognitive behavioral therapy for insomnia (CBT-I) is a multicomponent treatment, and not all people with sleep difficulties need all components. You may also remember that we often add elements of another treatment, called acceptance and commitment therapy (ACT), to help our clients get even better results. Not all people need these strategies, either. In this chapter we will help you use your sleep logs and the other assessments from chapter 1 to choose the treatment elements most suited to your particular "flavor" of sleep problem. We will also help you decide where to start. This will be a bit like a "choose your own adventure" book: you will jump around between chapters depending on your specific needs.

Let's start with an overview of the different types of strategies that make up our hybrid CBT-ACT treatment for insomnia. First, there are *behavioral strategies*. These form the backbone of CBT-I. We almost certainly will suggest that you use one of two behavioral programs—*stimulus control* (chapter 6) or *sleep restriction* (chapter 7)—or their combination (chapter 8). These are the two treatment components that we think are most essential. *Sleep hygiene* (chapter 9) is another behavioral treatment that you might add to stimulus control or sleep restriction.

Second, there are *cognitive strategies*, or strategies to work with the thoughts, attitudes, and beliefs that may be adding to your insomnia spiral. Dr. Allison Harvey and her collaborators (2014) have found that adding cognitive therapy to the behavioral treatment of insomnia leads to better results. We can help you identify and change thoughts that may be feeding your insomnia using something called *cognitive restructuring* (chapter 10). We can help you move sleep-interfering thought patterns—such as worrying, problem-solving, or planning—from the bedroom and bedtime to a different place and time during the day, using something called *designated worry time*, or DWT (chapter 11). And we can help you step back from your active mind and decrease what is called "cognitive hyperarousal" using strategies from ACT, such as *mindfulness* and *cognitive defusion* (chapter 12). You may benefit from all of these strategies. However, we will help you prioritize so you can learn really well one or two skills for working with your thoughts, instead of spreading your resources too thin.

As you read in the previous chapter, *willingness* (or *acceptance*) is another strategy from ACT that we make extensive use of. A small minority of our patients tell us that they are not worked up about their sleep. Most come back after a couple of weeks saying that they are becoming more aware of their stress or anxiety about sleep! So nearly everyone we have worked with ultimately benefits from acceptance strategies, which is part of the reason we put this so early in the book. Plus, for the behavioral programs to work, you need to be willing to do them—and do them fully.

We will be encouraging you to start with your core behavioral program (stimulus control therapy [SCT] and/or sleep restriction therapy [SRT]). If, by the end of this chapter, you are not willing to do this, then we will ask you to read about both treatments in case more information makes you more willing. If you still are not willing, you will start with cognitive strategies.

We will cover a lot of ground in this chapter. Here is our itinerary:

- You will decide if you will start by treating insomnia or another sleep disorder.

- We will guide you in making sense of all the information you collected in your sleep logs.

- You will choose a behavioral program.

- You will choose one or more cognitive strategies.

- We will address questions you may have about your use of sleep aids, such as medications or herbal remedies.

Worksheet 5.1 will help you pull together the work you do to create your personalized treatment plan. Fill it out one section at a time as you read the relevant section of this chapter. Remember to keep collecting data with your sleep log as you work through this chapter. Let's get started planning your adventure!

WORKSHEET 5.1: My Personalized Treatment Plan

Use this worksheet to pull together the work you'll do with exercises 5.1 and 5.2, and tables 5.1 and 5.2. This will help you get started and stay on track.

My First Step Will Be:

_____ Consulting a medical professional

_____ Treating a circadian rhythm disorder (appendix A)

_____ Treating insomnia (chapters 6–14)

My Destination (Treatment Goals)

Carefully consider where you want your adventure to take you. Be specific. Be realistic.

I hope to: _____ sleep more (_____ hours of sleep on a typical night)

_____ fall asleep more quickly (within _____ minutes of lights out)

_____ have fewer awakenings (no more than _____ per night)

_____ not wake too early (sleep until at least _____:_____)

_____ have less fitful/more restorative sleep

_____ be in bed less/have fewer hours dedicated to sleeping (no more than _____ hours between bedtime and final wake time)

_____ be less anxious about sleep

_____ have fewer daytime consequences of sleep

My Insomnia Program Road Map

I am going to start with this core behavioral treatment program:

_____ Stimulus control therapy (chapter 6)

_____ Sleep restriction therapy (chapter 7)

_____ Combined stimulus control and sleep restriction therapy (chapter 8)

I also will work on my sleep hygiene:

_____ Yes, I will read chapter 9 and consider whether there are some changes worth making.

_____ No, I have good sleep hygiene and do not want to put energy here.

These are the cognitive treatment strategies I plan to learn and practice. (Note: If you plan to use more than two, mark with an asterisk (*) the one or two strategies that you will focus on first.)

_____ Increasing willingness/decreasing struggle (chapter 4)

_____ Cognitive restructuring (chapter 10)

_____ Designated worry time (chapter 11)

_____ Cognitive defusion (chapter 12)

_____ Mindfulness (chapter 12)

Here is what I plan to do about the sleep aids (such as medications or herbs) that I currently use:

Aid	Keep Using	Stop Using			Consult Doctor
		Before	During	After	

Is Insomnia the Right Place to Start?

Complete exercise 5.1 using the work you did in chapter 1. This decision tree (a method of narrowing down your choices) will help you decide if you should start by treating insomnia. For each box, circle "yes" or "no" and follow the related branch. To summarize, if you are excessively sleepy during the day *and* you answered yes to a number of the screening questions for sleep apnea, restless legs syndrome (RLS), or periodic limb movement disorder (PLMD), we suggest that you start with a visit to a medical doctor to see if you should have a sleep study. If you are an extreme "night owl" or "morning lark," we suggest that you first work on this circadian rhythm issue. If you start with a medical consultation and do not have a neurological condition that needs medical treatment, we ask you to return here to treat your sleep problems. If you treat either a neurological condition or a circadian rhythm issue and continue to have insomnia, we also suggest you return here. If you treat a neurological condition or circadian rhythm issue and are sleeping well, congratulations! You can donate this book to someone who still is not sleeping well!

EXERCISE 5.1: Are you treating insomnia or something else?

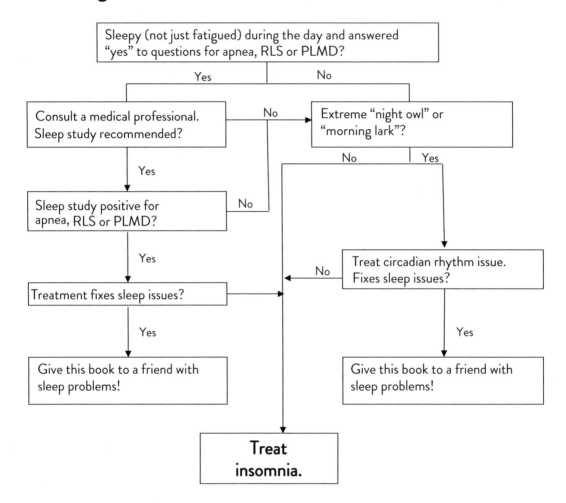

Your Insomnia Snapshot

Once you have two weeks of sleep log data, we encourage you to start a Sleep Log Summary. On worksheet 5.2 you can record your weekly averages for:

- Hours Asleep

- Time (Hours) in Bed

- Sleep Efficiency

Each of these numbers can be lifted right off of your sleep log. Although this may seem redundant, we find it quite helpful. By tracking your weekly averages over time, the worksheet will help you focus on overall patterns and trends. It is all too easy to hyperfocus on some particular night of sleep. This tends to be counterproductive, especially if your mind keeps focusing on your worst nights!

If you are a numbers person, and really like data, then the expanded version of the Sleep Log Summary in worksheet 5.3 may be the one for you. This worksheet guides you in pulling out from your sleep log even more data. Instead of looking at three variables, you will calculate and record weekly averages for seven. If we were treating you, we would be paying attention to all of the following variables to get a more complete picture of your sleep pattern:

- Sleep onset latency (SOL): this is how long it takes you to fall asleep in the beginning of the night. Specifically, SOL is the number of minutes between "lights out" (your asterisk or first down-arrow) and when you fall asleep (the start of your first solid or squiggly line).

- Wake after sleep onset (WASO): this is the number of minutes you are awake in the middle of the night—after you first fall asleep, but before your final awakening. On your sleep log, WASO is pictured as gaps or breaks in the lines that show when you were asleep.

- Awakenings: the number of times you wake up between sleep onset and your final awakening. This is a count of the number of vertical lines on your sleep log. Do not count your final awakening.

- Fatigue: calculating your average fatigue rating will help you focus on your daytime functioning and not just your nighttime sleep. It also will help you test any predictions you may have about how the treatment will make you feel during the day. For example, many people fear that they will be much more tired if they do either SCT or SRT. Some are and some are not.

For each of these variables, calculate your weekly average. That is, add your SOL for each night of the week, then divide the total by the number of nights for which you have data. Then do the same for WASO, awakenings, and fatigue.

Whichever format you choose, we encourage you to complete the Sleep Log Summary throughout your treatment program to help you track your progress. If you do not care to do this, please still complete it now for a pretreatment "snapshot." We will ask you in chapter 13 to again complete it for a couple of weeks. This will allow you to compare your insomnia before and after the treatment program.

WORKSHEET 5.2: **Sleep Log Summary (Simple)**

Treatment(s)	Week	Start Date	Average		
			Hours Asleep	Hours in Bed	Sleep Efficiency
(Pretreatment)	1				
(Pretreatment)	2				
	3				
	4				
	5				
	6				
	7				
	8				
	9				
	10				
	11				
	12				
	13				
	14				
	15				
	16				

Sample

Treatment(s)	Week	Start Date	Average		
			Hours Asleep	Hours in Bed	Sleep Efficiency
(Pretreatment)	1	08/06/15	5.5	7.1	77.5%
(Pretreatment)	2	08/13/15	5.75	9	63.9%
Drop the rope! Lean in.	3	08/20/15	5.5	8	68.8%
SRT 6 hrs. Bedtime routine.	4	08/27/15	5.5	6	91.7%
SRT (6.25). Add DWT.	5	09/03/15	6	6.25	96.0%
SRT (6.5). Add mindfulness.	6	09/10/15	5.8	6.5	89.2%
SRT (6.5–6.75). Add defusion.	7	09/17/15	6.25	6.65	94.0%
SRT (6.75–7).	8	09/24/15	6.75	6.93	97.4%
SRT (7–7.25). Stopped DWT.	9	10/01/15	6.75	7.18	94.0%

WORKSHEET 5.3: Sleep Log Summary (Expanded)

			Average						
Treatment(s)	Week	Start Date	Hours Asleep	Hours in Bed	Sleep Efficiency	SOL (min)	WASO (min)	Awakenings	Fatigue
(Pretreatment)	1								
(Pretreatment)	2								
	3								
	4								
	5								
	6								
	7								
	8								

Treatment(s)	Week	Start Date	Hours Asleep	Hours in Bed	Sleep Efficiency	SOL (min)	WASO (min)	Awakenings	Fatigue
	9								
	10								
	11								
	12								
	13								
	14								
	15								
	16								

Average

Sample

Week	Start Date	Hours Asleep	Hours in Bed	Sleep Efficiency	Average					Treatment(s)
					SOL (min)	WASO (min)	Awakenings	Fatigue		
1	08/06/15	5.5	7.1	77.5%	10	86	1	7.8		(Pretreatment)
2	08/13/15	5.75	9	63.9%	65	130	2.5	6.7		(Pretreatment)
3	08/20/15	5.5	8	68.8%	30	120	1	5.3		Drop the rope! Lean in.
4	08/27/15	5.5	6	91.7%	15	15	0.25	7.5		SRT 6 hrs. Bedtime routine.
5	09/03/15	6	6.25	96.0%	15	0	1	7.3		SRT (6.25). Add DWT.
6	09/10/15	5.8	6.5	89.2%	45	0	0	5.8		SRT (6.5). Add mindfulness.
7	09/17/15	6.25	6.65	94.0%	25	0	0	4.2		SRT (6.5–6.75). Add defusion.
8	09/24/15	6.75	6.93	97.4%	5	5.7	0.25	4.1		SRT (6.75–7).
9	10/01/15	6.75	7.18	94.0%	18	7.7	0.14	2.6		SRT (7–7.25). Stopped DWT.

Now, take a few moments to complete the first two sections of worksheet 5.1. What will your first step be? Where do you want to end up? Use your insomnia snapshot to think about how you want your sleep to be different. Set specific goals.

Your Insomnia Treatment Program

When we meet with clients, we use their data and their preferences to help them build an individualized treatment program that has a high likelihood of success. In this section we will help you do the same.

Choosing a Behavioral Treatment Program

Both stimulus control and sleep restriction are highly successful, both according to research and in our own clinical experience. Some clinicians who provide CBT-I always combine the two. We are in favor of this *if* you are completely willing and able to use a combined approach *and* there are not significant risks. However, many of our clients are not willing or able to do "the full shebang." We firmly believe that doing one treatment program fully works better than doing two "watered-down" programs. Plus, you may respond to just one of the programs, so doing a combined program may be a bigger "dose" of treatment than you need.

So where should you start? You should know up front that, nine times out of ten, we think either program will work equally well. In these cases we help people pick the one that they are most willing to do. However, your sleep pattern or sleep-related behaviors may lead us to recommend one treatment over the other.

You should also know that many people we work with start out being unwilling to do one of the programs, and then become willing once they understand the treatment rationale and how successful the program is. Many think they will hate a certain aspect of the program (such as getting up earlier) and then actually really like it. We will address many of these issues when we discuss each program in depth in the next two chapters. For now, feel free to use your initial instinct about which you are more willing to do to help you select where to start.

To help you decide which program to use, carefully review table 5.1, which compares and contrasts the two treatment programs and their combination.

TABLE 5.1: A Comparison of Stimulus Control, Sleep Restriction, and Their Combination

	Stimulus Control	Sleep Restriction	Combination
What you do (simplified)	Go to bed when sleepy. If you are awake in bed for more than twenty minutes at any point during the night, leave the bedroom. Return to bed when sleepy. Repeat as needed. Have a consistent wake time, no matter how much you slept. No daytime naps.	Limit your time in bed to the number of hours you are currently sleeping. Increase your time in bed by fifteen minutes after a week of sleeping 90% of the time you are in bed. Have a consistent sleep schedule. No daytime naps.	Limit your time in bed to the number of hours you are currently sleeping AND leave the bed if you are not sleeping. Have a consistent sleep schedule. No daytime naps.
Can be used with these sleep patterns	Awake for stretches of time when first going to sleep, in the middle of the night, and/or because waking too early.	Awake for stretches of time when first going to sleep, in the middle of the night, and/or because waking too early. Sleep is fitful, restless, or unrefreshing, but you aren't actually awake for any stretch of time. Multiple very brief awakenings.	Awake for stretches of time when first going to sleep, in the middle of the night, and/or because waking too early. May also have fitful sleep or many brief awakenings.
The program is especially well suited if you...	...sleep better away from your own bedroom; ...feel yourself getting tense or anxious as you approach bed; and/or ...do things in your bedroom other than sleep and have sex (like read, watch TV).	...are in bed for much more time than you are sleeping (for example, if you are sleeping less than 85% of the time you are in bed).	...want to be aggressive and are willing to do both programs (fully) at the same time.

	Stimulus Control	Sleep Restriction	Combination
You should *not* do the program (or should not do it without the help of an experienced professional) if you...	...have balance issues, a medical condition, or medications that put you at risk for falling if you leave the bed at night; ...have an injury or mobility issue that makes it hard to get in and out of bed multiple times; ...use CPAP or a similar device and have a hard time putting it on or getting settled with it.	...have a bipolar mood disorder, seizure disorder, or other medical condition that is made worse by too little rest.	...have any of the factors that suggest you should not do one of the programs.
What you may like about this program	You can have a full night's sleep if you happen to have a "good" night. You will not be lying in bed awake for long stretches of time.	Once in bed you can stay there and rest even if you are not sleeping. You do not have to make any decisions about when to get in and out of bed. You regain hours of your life to do things other than "try to sleep."	You will not be lying in bed awake for long stretches of time. You regain hours of your life to do things other than "try to sleep." Aggressive treatment may lead to quicker results.
What may be uncomfortable about this program	Making decisions about whether you have been awake long enough to get out of bed. Leaving the comfort of your bed/bedroom. Disturbing your bed partner or housemates by getting up and down.	Giving up the occasional night of adequate sleep you may be getting. Being awake and out of bed when you are exhausted.	You may have fewer hours in bed resting than with either program on its own.

Now take a look at your sleep log data. Do you have stretches of time in bed when you are awake for at least thirty minutes? Do you have fitful or restless sleep (indicated by wavy lines on your sleep log) or lots of brief awakenings during the night (indicated by horizontal lines)? Is your "sleep efficiency" (the amount of time in bed that you are asleep) under 85%? Use this information to work through exercise 5.2. For each box, circle "yes" or "no" and follow the related branch. Use this decision tree and the information in the table above to help you choose stimulus control therapy, sleep restriction therapy, or their combination. Record your choice on worksheet 5.1.

Now consider whether to add sleep hygiene to whichever core behavioral program you choose. You probably have seen sleep hygiene guidelines in popular media. If you are reading this book, chances are good that you have already addressed this "low-hanging fruit." Sleep hygiene alone is not likely to give you the restorative sleep you are seeking. However, having your behaviors in line with the sleep hygiene recommendations may help the other programs work better. That is why we suggest you add sleep hygiene to stimulus control and/or sleep restriction, rather than using it as a stand-alone treatment.

Again, look at your sleep log data: do you consume caffeine, nicotine, or alcohol? Do you exercise right before bed, or not at all? Think about your sleeping environment: is your room too cold or too hot? Too light? Too noisy or too quiet? Is your mattress uncomfortable, or do you sleep in a chair? Do pets or people disturb your sleep? Consider the hour before you retire: do you go, go, go right up until bedtime? Do you use electronic devices or have bright lights on? If you answered yes to any of the above, we suggest you read chapter 9 to learn more about how these behaviors and environmental conditions can interfere with sleep. Then you can decide if it is worth making some changes. Go ahead and mark worksheet 5.1 with your decision about whether you will read this chapter.

EXERCISE 5.2: Should you use stimulus control, sleep restriction, or both?

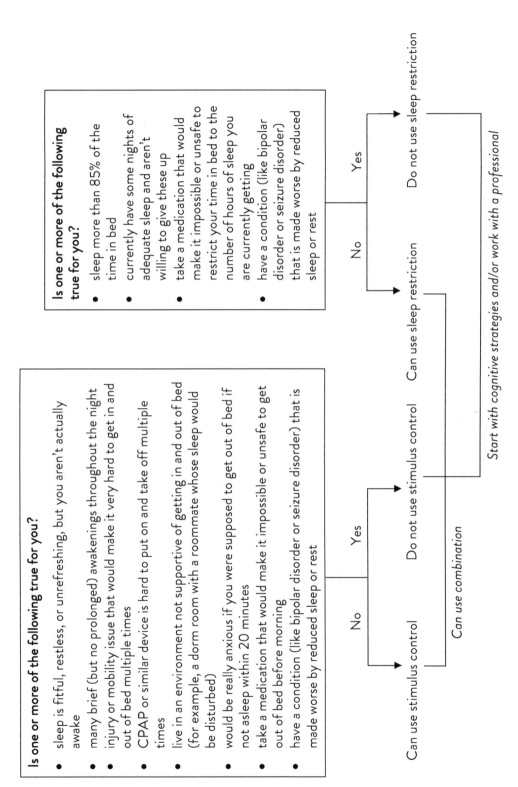

Is one or more of the following true for you?

- sleep is fitful, restless, or unrefreshing, but you aren't actually awake
- many brief (but no prolonged) awakenings throughout the night
- injury or mobility issue that would make it very hard to get in and out of bed multiple times
- CPAP or similar device is hard to put on and take off multiple times
- live in an environment not supportive of getting in and out of bed (for example, a dorm room with a roommate whose sleep would be disturbed)
- would be really anxious if you were supposed to get out of bed if not asleep within 20 minutes
- take a medication that would make it impossible or unsafe to get out of bed before morning
- have a condition (like bipolar disorder or seizure disorder) that is made worse by reduced sleep or rest

No → Can use stimulus control

Yes → Do not use stimulus control

Can use combination

Is one or more of the following true for you?

- sleep more than 85% of the time in bed
- currently have some nights of adequate sleep and aren't willing to give these up
- take a medication that would make it impossible or unsafe to restrict your time in bed to the number of hours of sleep you are currently getting
- have a condition (like bipolar disorder or seizure disorder) that is made worse by reduced sleep or rest

No → Can use sleep restriction

Yes → Do not use sleep restriction

Start with cognitive strategies and/or work with a professional

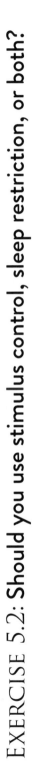

65

Alternative Routes for Your Next Step

There are four reasonable paths to take at this juncture.

1. If you are eager to get started, you can skip ahead to the chapter or chapters related to the behavioral treatment program you selected. Once your behavioral program is under way, return here to build your plan for working with your thoughts.

2. Alternatively, you can finish working through this chapter and complete worksheet 5.1 before launching your behavioral program.

3. If you are not willing to do either behavioral program, you can jump to chapters 6 and 7 to learn more about each. If this helps you become willing, you can return here to continue to develop your plan using worksheet 5.1.

4. If you are still unwilling to start SCT or SRT, continue to work through this chapter. You will start treatment with cognitive strategies. You may want to work specifically on the thoughts that are getting in the way of doing the behavioral treatment. These usually are some variation of *I do not want to, I am too scared to*, or *Why bother? Nothing will help.*

Choosing Cognitive Treatment Strategies

As explained in chapter 3, the way you think can impact your physiological arousal, which can affect your ability to sleep. Sometimes the *content* of your thoughts, or *what* you are thinking, increases arousal (for example, *If I do not sleep well tonight I'll be absolutely miserable tomorrow. I cannot stand another day like that!*). Other times, it is the *process* of thinking that interferes with sleep. That is, regardless of what you are thinking about, having a busy mind is likely to increase arousal and interfere with sleep. Here is a brief summary of the strategies we review in chapters 4 and 10–12 that may help you shift your thinking, facilitating a better night's sleep.

TABLE 5.2: Summary of Cognitive Strategies

Strategy	Description	Target	Helps most with...
Cognitive Restructuring (chapter 10)	Identify and challenge thoughts that are not fully true (for example, *I cannot stand another day of exhaustion*; or *Everyone needs eight hours of sleep*). Identify and modify thoughts that are unhelpful (*If I fall asleep now, I'll get six hours of sleep...if I fall asleep now, I'll get five hours...*)	Thought content	...correcting myths about "normal" sleep. ...catastrophic thoughts about what will happen if you do not sleep. ...thoughts that interfere with willingness to change behaviors. ...negative thoughts about other things in your life that increase stress or anxiety and (therefore) physiological arousal.
Designated Worry Time (chapter 11)	Set aside time during the day to worry, worry, worry. At all other times (including while in bed), if you catch yourself worrying, remind yourself that you can worry during your designated time, and refocus on something else.	Thought process	...a busy or active mind while in bed. Although designed for worry, this strategy can be modified to target most thought processes (such as planning, problem-solving, or fantasizing).
Mindfulness Practice (chapter 12)	Practice paying attention on purpose, in the present moment, and without judgment.	Thought process	...a busy or active mind while in bed. ...high stress or anxiety (and, therefore, physiological arousal) any time of day.

Strategy	Description	Target	Helps most with...
Defusion Strategies (chapter 12)	Learn to step back from your thoughts and hold them less tightly. Examples: picture your thoughts on the tickertape at the bottom of a TV screen, or floating away in balloons; sing your thoughts; speak thoughts in a funny voice (for example, Donald Duck); thank your mind for the thought (*Thanks, mind!*).	Thought process	...a busy or active mind while in bed. ...catastrophic thoughts about what will happen if you do not sleep. ...thoughts that interfere with willingness to change behaviors.
Acceptance/ Willingness Strategies (chapter 4)	Decrease arousal by accepting what is, rather than struggling against it. Take more effective action by being more willing to have uncomfortable sensations and emotions.	Thought content and thought process	...thoughts about how you will sleep tonight. ...thoughts about the consequences of insomnia. ...hesitancy or resistance to doing some or all of the treatment program. ...struggle against other things in your life (which creates more physiological arousal).

As already mentioned, you may benefit from all of these strategies, and you are welcome to work through the chapters in sequence. As psychologists, we have a mental map of which strategies we suggest for whom. If you prefer to focus your attention on one area, here are some things that would cause us to suggest that you start with a particular strategy if you were sitting in our office.

If you are very anxious about how your sleep will be each night, or if you are deeply fearful that your sleep problems will lead to dire consequences (for example, that you will lose your job, default on your mortgage, and have to live on the streets), then we would often start with (1) cognitive restructuring, and (2) acceptance strategies. We would coach you to use cognitive restructuring during the day in order to examine more closely your catastrophic thinking about your sleep. Once you are in bed, we would coach you to practice acceptance by "dropping the rope" and relaxing into whatever this night brings.

If you are lying awake for stretches of time and your mind is busy—with fantasy, worry, problem-solving, or planning—we would start with designated worry time.

If you are not really sure what you are thinking about sleep or what your mind is doing at night, we would help you become more aware using mindfulness.

If you have very strong beliefs about why treatment will not work or why you cannot do the treatment as described, we would probably start with defusion, although cognitive restructuring may be an equally good option.

Based on everything you have just read, which cognitive strategies will you include in your treatment program? With which will you start? Record your plan on worksheet 5.1.

What to Do About Medications or Herbal Remedies That You Take for Sleep

If you are not currently using any sleep aids, you can skip this section and pour your energy into your behavioral program and one or more cognitive strategies. But what if you are using sleep aids? By "sleep aids" we mean anything you put into your body that is intended to help you sleep. This includes things you can buy with or without a prescription. It includes things that are "natural" (such as melatonin, chamomile, or marijuana) or manufactured (such as Ambien [zolpidem], Lunesta [eszopiclone], trazodone, or Seroquel). We are going to use the term "sleep aid" instead of "medication" because many people only think of prescription pharmaceuticals or their over-the-counter counterparts (such as Unisom or Benadryl) when we say "medication."

Let's face it: you would not be reading this book if you were perfectly happy to use sleep aids and they were working fully and not causing unpleasant or unsafe side effects. Or to put it another way, you are either wanting to add CBT-I to your sleep aids for even more improvement, or you want to use fewer or no sleep aids. Here are some common questions that you may have, and our typical responses. Please keep in mind that we are not medical doctors. The information provided here is for educational purposes only, with the goal of helping you be a more informed consumer. Please consult with your physician before tinkering with medications in any way. Use worksheet 5.1 to jot down your thoughts about what you want to do with each sleep aid you use.

Can I do this treatment if I'm using sleep aids?

Yes, as long as you still experience symptoms of insomnia and the sleep aids do not interfere with your ability to follow the treatment guidelines (for example, being too groggy to get out of bed when you are supposed to). However, we sometimes think that sleep aids are actually making a person's sleep problem worse. For example, some sleep aids alter the architecture of sleep (that is, the structure and pattern of sleep). Others may increase your morning fatigue. This may worsen the daytime consequences of insomnia, or just make you think you slept more poorly than you did. If you have specific questions about how your sleep aids affect sleep architecture or other brain functions, consult your medical provider or pharmacist.

Sleep aids also can interfere with CBT-I. They may make you even less confident in your body's ability to sleep unassisted, feeding the very thinking we are trying to counter. On the other hand, you may have a lot less anxiety and physiological arousal just knowing that you have access to a sleep aid that works in the short term.

It is not about sleep aids being "right" or "wrong." It is about what works, not only tonight, but in the long run.

What should I expect if I stop using a sleep aid I've been using regularly?

If you stop a sleep aid you have been taking nightly, you may experience what we call "rebound insomnia"—an initial period of worsening of symptoms. The severity of symptoms may be even worse than before you started the sleep aid. We have witnessed rebound insomnia when people have come off of sedative hypnotics like zolpidem (Ambien) and eszopiclone (Lunesta), benzodiazepines like clonazepam (Klonopin) and lorazepam (Ativan), and marijuana. But we have also worked with people who have come off of these sleep aids and not had rebound insomnia.

The reason it is important to know about the potential for rebound is that the way you respond to any rebound symptoms can make a really big difference. If you think, *See, I really am dependent on that pill!* then you are likely to get right back on the sleep aid, and be distressed. If you have anxious thoughts like, *Oh no! Am I back to square one? Is this the start of a really awful period?* then you will feed into the insomnia spiral that we described in chapter 3. If, instead, you come off of a sleep aid *willing* (there's that word again!) to experience rebound symptoms, then you may stay off the sleep aid and be relaxed enough for your body to self-correct.

In general, you are less likely to experience rebound insomnia or uncomfortable withdrawal effects if you come off a sleep aid slowly, gradually decreasing the dose.

If I want to come off of sleep aids, should I do it before, during, or after my CBT-I program?

It depends. Some clinicians always wean patients off of sleep aids before starting CBT-I. There are some compelling reasons for approaching treatment this way. First, this approach ensures that you are treating your insomnia as it actually is, rather than how it is with sleep aids. For example, sometimes people tell us that they used to have trouble falling asleep; now, with a sleep aid, they fall asleep quickly but have lots of awakenings. Second, if you come off of sleep aids before CBT-I, you do not run the risk of rebound insomnia later, which could feel like a real setback after successful CBT-I. Third, the effects of the sleep aid may make it hard to follow the behavioral program guidelines. For example, you may wake up too groggy to get out of bed quickly. Finally, if the sleep aid is working well enough, you will not have the opportunity to use stimulus control therapy or sleep restriction therapy.

We generally recommend starting CBT-I even before coming off of sleep aids if you are very anxious about this change and want some specific tools in your toolbox first. We also encourage you to start CBT-I if you are coming off of a medication very slowly and do not want to wait months before getting additional help.

How should I use CBT-I if I am sleeping well now, but I want to stop using sleep aids?

First, we encourage you to hone cognitive skills now. If you do experience a sleep disruption, you can use these skills to respond in a way that does not feed the insomnia spiral. These skills also can help you manage concerns you have about stopping the sleep aids. We also encourage you to plan a behavioral treatment program: decide which strategies you will use, read the relevant chapters, and complete the related worksheets as fully as you can. This will allow you to respond quickly if insomnia does return after you stop the sleep aids.

Can I occasionally take something to get just one good night's sleep while I'm doing stimulus control or sleep restriction?

We encourage you not to do this except in the most extenuating of circumstances. Both programs rely, to some degree, on you consistently getting less sleep in order to build your sleep drive (see chapter 2). What we consider to be "extenuating circumstances" is different for different people. It will depend on your medical and mental health history, as well as your current roles and responsibilities.

I'm using melatonin and do not want to stop. What's the best way to take it?

Melatonin is a hormone that your body naturally releases as the sun goes down. It sets in motion a cascade of events that tells your brain when to sleep. Melatonin levels remain high throughout the night. Your body then stops releasing it during the day.

There is widespread disagreement about whether melatonin supplements help, hurt, or have no impact on insomnia. Some clinicians think it is fine to take melatonin any time of night, since it is normal to have high levels of melatonin throughout the night. Others believe that an increase in melatonin well after sunset (for example, at bedtime or in the middle of the night) will confuse your body clock and throw off your circadian rhythm. These clinicians suggest taking melatonin earlier than most people take it, such as between 7 and 9 p.m.

There is greater agreement that properly timed melatonin can help treat sleep issues related to shift work, jet lag, and circadian rhythm problems. If you do take melatonin supplements, the sleep physicians we work with suggest lower doses (0.3–3 mg) than many of our clients report taking.

What if I take a medication for another medical condition?

Some medications that are prescribed for insomnia may also be prescribed for something else. For example, trazodone may be prescribed for depression, quetiapine (Seroquel) may be prescribed for bipolar disorder or psychosis, and a benzodiazepine may be prescribed for anxiety. This is one reason we ask you to consult your physician before making any changes to your sleep aids—we do not want you to unknowingly stop treatment for a different condition.

Some medications may be contributing to your insomnia. For example, stimulating medications like Wellbutrin (bupropion), Adderall (dextroamphetamine/amphetamine), and decongestants (like pseudoephedrine) can interfere with sleep if taken too late in the day. If you take any medications, you may want to ask a pharmacist if any of them could be contributing to your sleep problems. Then talk to your physician about whether taking the medication at a different time or dose might be helpful.

What about medical (or recreational) marijuana?

Like any sleep aid, marijuana can mask your actual sleep pattern, interfere with your ability to implement CBT-I fully, stop working over time, and create rebound insomnia when you decrease or stop use.

Your Next Step

At this point in the program, you have some basic education about how sleep works, how your behaviors and thoughts can maintain sleep problems over time, and how CBT-I can help you change your behaviors and thoughts to restore your sleep (and your relationship with sleep). You have either determined that you should start by treating insomnia, or you diverted from this program to treat a neurological condition (such as sleep apnea) or a circadian rhythm disorder, and have returned here because you also have insomnia.

Hopefully you have continued to keep a sleep log. You have been practicing being willing to not sleep, accepting whatever this particular night brings. You have worked through the exercises in this chapter and you have created your personalized treatment plan. If you are willing to do whichever behavioral program you landed on, you will now proceed to the relevant chapter or chapters and start your program! Once you have started, you will start reading about and practicing the cognitive strategies that are part of your program.

If you are not ready to start a behavioral program, we invite you to read the next two chapters to see if more detailed information increases your willingness. If it does, you will start your behavioral program and then move on to cognitive strategies. If it does not, you will start with cognitive strategies, specifically targeting those thoughts and feelings that are keeping you from doing a behavioral program. If you are still stuck, consider using this book with the help of a trained professional, or with a "buddy" in your life who also has sleep difficulties.

Finally, if you have been using sleep aids, you may continue to use them, or you may decide to decrease or discontinue your use of them either before, during, or after the program. You may want to consult a professional to decide which timing is best for you, or for help with how to taper off of the sleep aids.

Ready? Let's go!

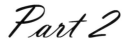

Part 2

BEHAVIORAL
STRATEGIES

*T*his section is dedicated to the behavioral treatments that form the backbone of cognitive behavioral therapy for insomnia. In each chapter we strive to hold your hand just as we would if you were our client. We will help you understand the rationale for the challenging program you are about to start. We will give you very detailed instructions. We will answer the most common questions clients ask us. We will help you anticipate and troubleshoot potential roadblocks. And we will continually remind you to track your progress.

Behavioral change is hard in the best of circumstances, and you may be worn down from months or years or even decades of insomnia. The treatments included in this section do require hard work. They may make you feel even more tired at first. And they work. We would not ask you to do this hard work or take on this discomfort if we had not witnessed the dramatic improvements our clients have had. Nor would we ask you to do this hard work if we knew of an easier, more comfortable way.

We want you to think of this part of your sleep adventure as "working a program." We are not asking you to commit to these behavioral changes forever. It is enough to commit for right now. In chapter 14 we will help you figure out when and how to phase out your behavioral sleep program.

Look back at the treatment plan you developed using worksheet 5.1. Did you select stimulus control therapy, sleep restriction therapy, or the combination as your core behavioral treatment program? Go ahead and jump to the related chapter now.

Chapter 6

Retrain Your Brain (Stimulus Control Therapy)

*L*et's take a typical person who is sleeping really well. Say she averages eight hours of sleep each night, and likes to read in bed until her eyes become so heavy she cannot read anymore, usually about thirty minutes. She turns out the lights and falls asleep quickly; she sleeps through the night with no awakenings, except perhaps getting up for a minute to go to the bathroom. She is in bed eight and a half hours, and sleeps for eight, which means she is sleeping 94% of the time that she is in bed. Because of this, her brain very strongly associates the bed with sleep. She can afford to do something else in bed (read) without disturbing her sleep, because over 90% of the time she is in bed, she is sleeping. At an unconscious level, her brain knows: *bed = sleep.* When she gets into bed at night, her brain starts to prepare for sleep. What else would it do? The bed is for sleep, right?

Now let's say this same woman has some stressful life changes and no longer falls asleep quickly when she turns out the lights. Instead, her mind gets busy: *Will I do okay in this new job position? What if they decide it was a mistake to promote me? How will Tom and the kids handle the fact that I'm working more hours? Melissa is really starting to struggle in school. How will I stay on top of that when I'm working more? Am I being a bad mom? I am a bad mom. Like yesterday—why did I yell at Ryan? He wasn't really doing anything so wrong....* And on and on her mind chatters as she tries to fall asleep. Now she is only sleeping about six hours each night. By nighttime she is exhausted, so she starts to go to bed earlier, hoping to catch more sleep. Instead of being in bed for eight and a half hours, she is in bed nine, and then, as time goes on, nine and a half hours. She does get a little more sleep, but still only about six and a half hours. Now she is only sleeping 68%, or two-thirds, of the time that she is in bed. And not only does she read and sleep in bed, she also worries and lies awake in bed. Bed no longer equals sleep. Bed = sleep or reading or worrying or lying awake. When she gets into bed at night, her brain does not automatically prepare for sleep. Why should it? It may be time to read or worry or just lie there, rather than sleep. Over time, her sleep problems may get even worse. When she wakes in the middle of the night to go to the bathroom, her mind may get activated when she climbs back into bed. Now she not only has trouble falling asleep in the beginning of the night, but also has long awakenings in the middle of the night.

Stimulus control therapy (SCT) is a program that can help you retrain your brain to strongly pair bed with sleep. To do this, we want to minimize the link between bed and everything else, including other activities (such as reading or watching television) and internal states of arousal (such as frustration, stress, fear, or worry). You want to give your brain and body a smaller menu of options when you hit the bed. We also want to weaken the association between sleep and everywhere other than bed. That is, you will use your bed only for sleep and sex, and you will sleep only in bed. SCT was the first behavioral program developed to treat insomnia (Bootzin & Perlis, 2011), and we know both from our clinical experience and from well-controlled research studies that it works (Morin et al., 2006).

Who Should Use Stimulus Control Therapy?

As we said in chapter 5, both stimulus control and sleep restriction are likely to work for you, so we usually suggest picking the one you are most willing to do fully. However, sometimes one treatment is a better fit, based on your sleep pattern. Here are some clues that SCT is likely to work well for you:

- Your insomnia takes the form of long periods of being awake, either in the beginning, middle, or end of the night.

- You stay in bed when you cannot sleep, or use the bed or bedroom for things other than sleep and sex.

- You sleep in places other than your bed (such as a couch or a guest room).

- You get sleepy while you are in a different room, and then feel more alert or anxious when you get into bed.

- You sleep better away from home.

We suggest you start with sleep restriction instead of SCT if:

- Your sleep is fitful, restless, or unrefreshing, but you are not fully awake for stretches of time.

- You have many brief (but no prolonged) awakenings throughout the night.

- You take a medication or have a health condition that makes it difficult or unsafe for you to get out of bed in the middle of the night.

- You are simply unwilling to leave your bed, even after you have read about this roadblock later in this chapter.

Stimulus Control Therapy: Basic Recipe

1. Limit your behavior in bed and in your bedroom to sleep and sex.

2. Lie down only when you are sleepy.

3. If, at any time during the night, you are awake for more than twenty minutes, leave the bedroom and do something boring or relaxing.

4. Return to bed when you are sleepy. (Do not sleep in another room.)

5. Repeat steps 3–4 as needed.

6. Fix your wake time—get up at the same time each morning regardless of how much sleep you got.

7. No daytime naps.

Stimulus Control Therapy: Detailed Instructions

Let's take a much closer look at each step. Many times we meet people who think they have done SCT, but upon further questioning we learn they missed some of the nuances. In our experience, these nuances are important, so we want to hold your hand as much as possible to ensure that you have the best chance of benefiting from your SCT program!

1. Limit behavior in bed and in your bedroom to sleep and sex.

Remember, we want the bed to cue your brain to sleep, and only sleep. Take stock—what else do you do in your bed or bedroom? Do you watch TV? Use a smartphone, tablet, or computer? Read? Talk with your bed partner? Do work or pay bills? Do you lie in bed and ruminate (think about the past again, and again, and again), worry, plan, problem-solve, or fantasize?

If you answered yes to any of these, take some time to figure out where you can do these activities other than your bedroom. Designate a new "home" for your electronic devices. Pick a spot in another room where you can read, work, or pay bills. Use "designated worry time" (chapter 11) to move your thinking to another time and place. Why is sex allowed but nothing else? Bootzin and Perlis (2011, 24) explain that most of us are "just not very creative about where we have sex"!

2. Lie down only when sleepy.

This is a little more complicated than it sounds. We want you to go to bed when you are sleepy so that it is more likely that you will fall asleep quickly (remember, we're shooting for bed = sleep). However, a consistent bedtime does help. Therefore, we encourage you to pick a target bedtime, and set yourself up to be sleepy by that time each night: start to wind down about sixty minutes earlier and complete your bedtime routine (such as personal hygiene and changing into pajamas) as if you are going to get into bed at your target time. If you are sleepy, get into bed and turn out the lights. If you are not, stay out of the bedroom and do something that is likely to help you get sleepy, and go to bed once you are sleepy.

There is an exception to this guideline: some people do not feel sleepy until they lie down in a dark room. If this sounds like you, you can experiment by going to bed at your target bedtime each night, regardless of how sleepy you are. If you don't fall asleep within about twenty minutes, you will get up (see step 3).

3. If, at any time during the night, you are awake for more than twenty minutes, leave the bedroom and do something boring or relaxing.

The original instructions for SCT state that you should leave the bed if you are awake for ten minutes (Bootzin & Perlis, 2011). We suggest that you leave the bedroom after twenty minutes to try to strike a balance. On the one hand, we want to limit the amount of time you are in bed awake. On the other hand, it is completely normal for it to take up to twenty minutes to fall asleep, and we don't want to set up unrealistic expectations. Given our primary goal of retraining your brain, you can absolutely get up sooner if you are so alert, annoyed, or anxious that you know sleep isn't coming anytime soon.

Here are a few additional pointers. Worksheet 6.1 guides you in establishing a specific plan for where you will go and what you will do if you are not sleeping.

- Don't watch the clock; check the time when you have the strong sense that it has been about twenty minutes. You will get better at estimating with practice.

- Plan ahead. Know where you will go and what you will do. Have materials ready.

- Use low lighting. If you are reading on a back-lit screen, dim it as much as possible and have no ambient light. Otherwise, use a lamp with a dim bulb (around twenty-five watts). Darkness signals to your brain that it's nighttime; light is stimulating. Some people suggest you not use anything with a screen (phone, electronic reader, computer) because of the light that screens emit. If you are not willing to avoid screens, consider wearing sunglasses that block out the blue rays of the light spectrum. These are readily available for purchase on the Internet.

- Choose activities that are boring or relaxing, not stimulating, such as folding laundry, ironing, knitting, reading, or listening to an audiobook or podcast. Pick things that you can put down at any time (such as uncomplicated knitting projects, magazines with short articles, books you have read before). If you choose to read or listen to something, pick material that does not get your mind too activated. This is different for everyone: some people can read work-related material while others cannot; some can read or listen to the news, while others get too distressed.

- Choose activities that do not make you overly productive. You do not want to do so much housework or work-related reading that your brain learns that nighttime is productive time.

- Anticipate and troubleshoot difficulties. For example, if it will be hard to get out of bed because the house will be cold, have a bathrobe and slippers beside your bed and a blanket where you will be sitting. If you know you'll be thirsty and the kitchen is a flight of stairs away, have water waiting for you.

4. Return to bed when you are sleepy. (Do not sleep in another room.)

There is no designated amount of time to stay out of bed. You may feel sleepy and return to bed after just a few minutes, or it may take hours, or it may not happen at all before your wake time. As soon as you notice yourself feeling sleepy, return to bed and give yourself up to twenty minutes to fall asleep.

Just like going to bed in the beginning of the night, there is one exception. If you know that you do not get sleepy until you lie down in a dark room, then you may want to return to bed after a set amount of time, such as twenty minutes.

Remember, part of strengthening the connection between bed and sleep is to sleep only in bed. Therefore, even if moving to the bedroom gets you more alert, in the long term SCT will work better if you don't fall asleep elsewhere.

5. Repeat steps 3–4 as needed.

On any given night, you may get up and go back to bed multiple times, once, or not at all.

6. Fix your wake time—get up at the same time each morning regardless of how much sleep you got.

We often say that if you are only willing to do one thing to help your sleep, have a consistent wake time. The importance of this step cannot be overstated!

Fixing your wake time will help you establish a regular sleep-wake rhythm, which supports healthy sleep and leads to less daytime sleepiness (Manber et al., 1996). Also, if you stay in bed later some mornings, fewer hours will have passed and your sleep drive will be lower at your target bedtime the next night, possibly making it harder to fall asleep quickly.

The standard SCT instructions do say that you can "sleep in" up to one hour later on non-work days (Bootzin & Perlis, 2011). We generally encourage you not to do this, so you can harness the full power of a consistent sleep-wake schedule. We are most likely to support a later rising time on non-work days if you (1) have to wake up earlier than your natural rhythm on work days, and (2) are getting significantly less sleep than you need (as opposed to cobbling together the right amount of sleep, but in disjointed fashion). In these cases, the extra hour of sleep two mornings a week can make you less tired, while your overall "sleep debt" will help you fall asleep at your target bedtime even after having slept in. If you try to sleep later on non-work days and notice that you sleep worse the next night, we encourage you to have a consistent wake time every day.

In setting your target bedtime and consistent wake time, we encourage you to choose times that give you a "sleep window" of no more than the total amount of sleep you think you need each night. For example, if you need eight hours of sleep, choose 10:30 p.m.–6:30 a.m., not 9:30 p.m.–7 a.m. Because you have come to expect to be awake in the middle of the night, it is natural to give yourself a larger sleep window. However, this tends to backfire, as you will see if you read about sleep restriction or the combination of SCT and SRT.

7. No daytime naps.

Naps deprive you of the opportunity to harness the power of sleep deprivation to help you fall asleep quickly and to stay asleep at night. Also, sleeping during the day may weaken the association between *nighttime* and sleep, which you want to strengthen. Finally, often when people nap during the day they do not do it in their beds. Remember, to strengthen the link between bed and sleep, you should sleep only in bed.

Common Questions (and Answers) or Roadblocks (and Possible Solutions)

"But I've always read in bed and I love it! Do I really have to give it up forever?"

First, you don't *have* to do anything. And telling yourself that you "have to" can actually get in the way. But you may *choose* to follow this guideline because you have hope that this method will work!

And, no, it does not have to be forever. We encourage people to think of it as "working a program." *Right now* you are doing stimulus control, and we encourage you to do it fully to give it the best chance of working. Once you are sleeping better, you may choose to go back to reading in bed. If you keep sleeping well, great! If your sleep starts to get worse, you probably will decide it is worth it to do your reading elsewhere. A lot of the people we have worked with have been surprised how easy it is to read or watch television (or do whatever they were doing in bed) somewhere else, and then move to the bed when it is time to sleep. You do not have to stop doing what you currently do right before bed. We are just suggesting you do it somewhere other than the bedroom.

"What's wrong with napping? Entire cultures revolve around a midday siesta!"

Just like the instruction to not read or do anything else in bed, we aren't asking you to give up naps forever. But napping during the day may weaken the connection between sleep and night. So while you are working a stimulus control program to treat your nighttime insomnia, we want you to sleep only at night. Also, you may remember from chapter 2 that your sleep drive will increase the longer you are awake, and will be partially discharged by any sleep you get; we want your sleep drive to be as high as possible at your target bedtime to facilitate falling asleep quickly.

"I have no place other than my bedroom."

We have worked with people who live in studio apartments and people who are trying to stick to stimulus control while staying at hotels. Although you will ideally use your bedroom only for sleep and sex, you can still do stimulus control even in the tightest of quarters. For example, one woman we worked with used one side of her queen-sized bed for reading and the other for sleeping! Others have gotten creative by setting up a cozy spot on the floor with some large pillows. One man who often travels got in the habit of looking for a chair on his floor of the hotel (he usually found one by the elevators); if he needed to leave his bed, he retreated to the chair with his book (and room key!). Another client padded the bathtub with blankets and pillows and read in there while her family slept in their shared hotel room on vacation.

"Even when I'm sleeping well it takes me thirty minutes to fall asleep. Should I still get up after twenty minutes?"

Most clinicians would suggest that you still get up within twenty minutes, thinking that any longer than that gives you too much time to associate bed with wakefulness. We have mixed feelings about this because we want to support your natural sleep rhythms and don't want to overpathologize it if you take thirty minutes to fall asleep. We generally suggest that people do an experiment and see what works. If you can be in bed for thirty minutes and not feel frustrated or anxious about the fact that you are not yet sleeping, then it may be reasonable to do this in the beginning of the night, but to give yourself less time to fall asleep if you wake in the middle of the night. On the other hand, we suggest you get up sooner if you are starting to get frustrated or anxious.

"I never really feel sleepy. When should I go (or return) to bed?" (Or: "Paying attention to whether I'm sleepy enough to return to bed is getting me more amped up. What should I do?")

If "sleepy" is a foreign concept to you, go to bed at your target bedtime in the beginning of the night. First, though, think carefully about whether that target bedtime is realistic given your natural sleep-wake (circadian) rhythm. If you know that you are a "night owl," we would suggest setting your bedtime after 10 p.m. even if you have to get up early for daytime obligations. If you start to sleep the entire time you are in bed but are not getting enough sleep, you can start to move your bedtime earlier in small increments, to see if you can adjust your clock (see appendix A for more information on shifting your clock).

Regarding when to return to bed after leaving it if you don't tend to feel sleepy or if you get anxious scanning your body for signs of sleepiness, consider using twenty minutes as a rule of thumb. You'll get out of bed again if it becomes clear that you are not going to fall asleep quickly.

"I'm exhausted all the time. What do you mean when you say I should go to bed when sleepy?"

Being tired or exhausted is different than being sleepy. By "sleepy" we mean that you feel as if you could fall asleep. Additional signs of sleepiness include yawning, heavy or droopy eyes, or head-nodding.

"Given how sleep deprived I am, shouldn't I rest in bed? Even if I'm not fully asleep, at least I'm not fully awake and alert either!"

If you rest in bed when not sleeping, you *may* feel better the next day, but this is a very short-term benefit, with the risk of feeding the insomnia spiral in the long term. Plus, most people we have worked with don't actually feel much better resting in bed; their minds just tell them that surely they will feel worse if they are spending less time in bed! You can use the fatigue ratings on your sleep log to look at the data and see if you do feel significantly better when you rest in bed. (However, see below for some information on why you may, indeed, feel worse when you first start SCT.)

"I'm fighting off a cold or flu. What should I do?"

Our bodies do need more rest when we are sick or getting sick. Try to give your body that rest while keeping the basic principles in place: rest on a couch or chair; sleep in bed. If you are sleeping a lot, you will be in bed a lot. If you need a lot of rest but can't sleep, you will be on the couch a lot.

"I don't look at the clock when I wake up in the middle of the night because it makes me anxious or alert. How will I know if I've been awake for twenty minutes?"

Although you can use your instinctive sense of how much time has passed, most people are not very accurate. We suggest having a stopwatch at the ready. When you awaken, reach out (ideally with eyes still closed) and start it. You can check it to see how much time has elapsed (without seeing the time) when you think it is time to leave the bed.

"I'm really enjoying spending less time in bed, and more time [reading, listening to podcasts, watching movies, being productive ...]. Is this a problem?"

It depends. If you are simply recapturing time when it is normal for you to be awake, celebrate your freedom from the tyranny of insomnia! Even if you are not yet sleeping better, at least you are giving up less for insomnia; it is having less control over your life. This is a wonderful thing! However, if you are really enjoying having a two-hour stretch in the middle of the night to have the house to yourself, do something relaxing, or get stuff done, then you may be training your brain to be awake during hours you want it to be asleep.

"I tend to eat if I'm up in the middle of the night. Is that okay?"

It is best not to train your body to expect food during your sleep period. Do your best to consume enough calories during the day that your body is not needing fuel overnight. This may mean having a small snack before bed (see chapter 9 for more about this). If you occasionally are too hungry to sleep, it will help to have a snack. However, try not to make this a habit.

"I just don't want to [give up other activities in bed; get out of bed if not sleeping]!"

You don't have to *want* to do a particular thing in order to do it. Try this exercise: say three times "I don't want to raise my arm." On the second time, start to raise your arm; have it fully in the air by the time you are done with the third round. Were you able to raise your arm even though your mind told you that you didn't want to? This may seem silly, but we encourage you to practice this throughout the day: say "I don't want to open the door" as you open it, or "I don't want to turn off the light" as you turn it off. (Similarly, if you think *I can't get out of bed*, do the same exercises saying "I *can't* raise my arm" and "I *can't* open the door.") Get practice doing things regardless of what your mind says about wanting or being able to do them. If you simply are not willing to follow the SCT guidelines, then you can consider sleep restriction. If this is not an option (based on the exercises in the last chapter, or because you aren't willing to do that either), then you can start with cognitive strategies, especially working with the thoughts that are interfering with your willingness to do the behavioral programs.

"I'm really worried that I'll be too tired to do what I have to do, or that getting less rest is dangerous to my health."

You may (or may not) feel worse before you feel better (see below). We encourage you to consider this possibility in your planning, both in terms of timing and for safety. For example, if you have a really important deadline or event next week, you may decide to wait to start this program until you are on the other side of it. If you are worried about whether it will be safe for you to drive, consider asking other people for rides, taking public transportation, or walking. If you work as a bus driver or a long-distance truck driver (for example), you may decide to start the program during a week off, to see if you are more sleepy and assess whether or not it is safe to work while doing the program.

"I'm trying to do the program, but sometimes I fall asleep on the couch [in the morning after my wake time, at midday, in the early evening]. I'm just so tired!"

We understand. Here are some things that have helped some of our clients stay awake when they aren't supposed to be sleeping: sit rather than reclining or lying down; hold a glass full of ice—you will get pretty quick feedback if you start to fall asleep; enlist the help of a housemate if someone else is up with you; if your eyes start to close, get up and leave the house (walk around the block, visit a friend) or do some jumping jacks or go up and down a flight of stairs.

What to Expect

You may be wondering how long it will take for this treatment to work. Your sleep may improve almost immediately: just knowing that there is a plan and that you won't be lying awake in bed for hours may give you tremendous relief, and with this relief will come decreased physical arousal and increased ability to sleep. Just having the plan is so powerful for some people that they rarely have to leave their bed. Or you may experience quick improvement simply because you have recaptured hours of your life that you had given over to insomnia. Even if you are not sleeping more, by being out of bed and spending more time doing enjoyable activities, you may feel a lot better.

For most people, though, improvement takes more time. The process of retraining your brain may take several weeks. The first few nights you will be adjusting to a new way of doing things, and you may even feel a little anxious about the treatment, so you may sleep even worse than usual. It is at this point that people often call us seeking some reassurance. Our general response is that it is normal to be anxious or worried, *and* we have very high confidence that the program will work if you do it fully and stick with it. We want to encourage you in this way, too.

You also may feel worse initially because you may actually get less sleep at first. Let's say you get out of bed because you are not sleeping and you return to bed thirty minutes later. It is possible that you would have fallen asleep in just five minutes if you had stayed in bed, in which case doing SCT cost you twenty-five minutes of sleep. Are you feeling anxious just reading this? We know it can be hard to risk precious minutes of sleep when you are struggling with chronic insomnia. Remember that you are reading this book because what you are currently doing is not working. Are you willing to experience more short-term pain for long-term gain? We don't say this flippantly. We know how hard it can be. We are asking you to do this hard work because we have seen people who have suffered the discomfort of insomnia for years or even decades have dramatic improvement when they were willing to feel even worse at first.

Whether you improve quickly or it takes weeks, your improvement may not be linear. You may "take two steps forward and one step back." Try this exercise: stand up, and pick a destination about ten feet from you. Take two steps toward your destination, then one step back toward where you started. If you keep doing this, where do you end up? It may not be as quick, and it may take more effort compared with constant forward motion, but you will still get to your destination if you persist.

How you respond to a setback can make all the difference in where you end up. If you respond with fear or extreme frustration, you will trigger more physical arousal and have a harder time getting back to sleep that night or getting to sleep the next night. You also may give up on the treatment program all together. This reaction to what could have been a temporary setback can get you stuck right back where you started. On the other hand, if you can practice acceptance and surrender to whatever this night brings (chapter 4) and stick with the program, there is a good chance the backward step will be followed by another two forward.

Your Stimulus Control Therapy Plan

Use worksheet 6.1 to develop your personalized SCT plan. Really think about each part of the plan. (Where will you go? What will you do?) Set yourself up for success by making the necessary preparations. After you complete the worksheet, ask yourself if you are willing to commit to the plan you just made. You need not commit for weeks. Are you willing to commit to your SCT plan for the next twenty-four hours?

WORKSHEET 6.1:
Your Stimulus Control Therapy Plan

Stimulus Control: Basic Recipe

1. Limit behavior in bed and in your bedroom to sleep and sex.

2. Lie down only when sleepy.

3. If, at any time during the night, you are awake for more than twenty minutes, leave the bedroom and do something boring or relaxing.

4. Return to bed when sleepy. (Do not sleep in another room.)

5. Repeat steps 3–4 as needed.

6. Fix your wake time—get up at the same time each morning regardless of how much sleep you got.

7. No daytime naps.

Where in my home I will go:

Activities I will engage in (*be specific!*):

Preparations to make ahead of time (for example, put low-watt bulb in table lamp, select book):

My target bedtime: _____   My consistent wake time: _____

Strategies for avoiding naps or nodding off:

What I will have to give up (for example, "the comfort of going to sleep to the sound of the TV," "the solitude I get from spending time in my room," "sleeping in on weekends"):

What discomfort I may experience (for example, "I may be even more tired at first," "I may be really sleepy without my afternoon nap or sleeping in on weekends," "Guilt for disturbing my bed partner"):

Why I'm willing to give these things up (for now) and experience these discomforts (for now):

Your Next Step

Once your SCT program is under way, you may want to start working on the other treatment elements that you selected on worksheet 5.1. But don't let that distract you from your SCT program: remember, we would rather you do one treatment component fully than do several parts of the treatment in watered-down fashion.

Continue to track your sleep by completing the sleep log each night. As instructed, use arrows to track when you get in and out of bed. This will help you evaluate how closely you are following the program. At the end of each week, calculate your average total sleep time, time in bed, and sleep efficiency. Also record your weekly averages on your Sleep Log Summary (worksheet 5.2 or 5.3), and use this worksheet to track when you start SCT and other parts of your treatment program.

How to Evaluate Your Progress and When to Consider a Different Plan

In chapter 13 we will help you thoroughly evaluate your treatment program after six to eight weeks. But you probably will want some feedback before then. Each week, take a few minutes to look at the data you are collecting. Is your total sleep time going up even a little bit compared with the weeks before you started the program? Is your sleep less fitful (are there more solid and fewer squiggly lines on your sleep log)? Are you falling asleep more quickly? Are you spending less time awake in the middle of the night? How are you feeling during the day?

We encourage you to stick with SCT for several weeks even if you are not seeing any obvious improvements. It can take some time for your brain to more readily pair bed and sleep. After all, it probably has had months or years of associating bed with insomnia! Research studies usually test a six-week treatment program, so do not give up too early. Also, you may get better results when you add to SCT other parts of your treatment program, such as cognitive strategies.

We also encourage you to look each week at how closely you are following the SCT instructions. Review the instructions and look closely at your sleep logs. Are there stretches of greater than twenty minutes when you are in bed awake? Do you have some notes indicating that you slept on the couch? Is your wake time consistent, or do you have days of sleeping in or going back to bed after your designated wake time? Are you engaging in activities that are stimulating and keeping you awake? We have been surprised how often people think they are doing the treatment when they actually are not following the guidelines very closely.

If your sleep is not improving, or not improving as quickly as you would like, the first thing we recommend is that you do the program even more fully, if there is any room at all for improvement. Are you willing to recommit to your SCT program?

If you follow SCT fully for three to four weeks and are seeing no benefit at all, then it may be time to switch to or add sleep restriction therapy. You also can consider switching to SRT if you are not willing to do SCT fully. If SRT is not a safe option for you, or if you also are unwilling to do that treatment, then you can turn your attention to cognitive strategies. Or this may be a good time to seek the support of a professional trained in CBT-I.

Are you ready to jump in? Good luck with this part of your adventure!

Chapter 7

Quality Over Quantity
(Sleep Restriction Therapy)

*Y*ou may remember from chapter 3 that what you do in response to poor sleep can greatly influence whether your sleep problems become chronic. One common response to unreliable sleep is to spend more and more time "trying" to sleep. You may stay in bed longer and longer. Or maybe there are more hours between your initial bedtime and final rise time, with stretches in the middle during which you are out of bed. Or perhaps you take naps during the day. You may be chasing more sleep every night of the week, or just on weekends. As you spend more time trying to sleep, your sleep thins out to cover the wider territory you set aside for it. You may experience this as light, fitful, or non-restorative sleep, or as multiple awakenings throughout the night. For example, if you are regularly getting six hours of sleep, you may say, "Yeah, but they're not even six *good* hours!"

In sleep restriction therapy (SRT) we limit your sleep window (the hours you set aside for sleep) to match the amount of sleep your body currently is getting. The result? Your sleep is likely to consolidate: it will knit back together and you will have fewer interruptions; your sleep will be deeper and more restful. At first you may still have all the daytime consequences of insomnia (such as fatigue or "foggy" thinking) because you still will not be getting enough sleep. However, once you have a stable base of consolidated sleep, we will build on that to get you back to a healthy amount of sleep.

Who Should Use Sleep Restriction Therapy?

As we said in chapter 5, both sleep restriction and stimulus control are likely to work for you, so we often suggest picking the one you are most willing to do fully. Having said that, we would recommend SRT over SCT if any of the following are true:

- Your sleep is fitful, restless, or unrefreshing, but you are not fully awake for stretches of time.

- You have many brief (but no prolonged) awakenings throughout the night.

- You are unable to do SCT because mobility issues make it unsafe to leave your bed if you are not sleeping.

We suggest you start with SCT instead of SRT if:

- You currently have some nights of adequate sleep and you are not willing to give these up.

- You are not willing to restrict your time in bed, even after you read about this roadblock later in this chapter.

Sleep Restriction Therapy: Basic Recipe

1. Calculate your average total sleep time (TST), average time in bed (TIB), and sleep efficiency (SE) using sleep log data for ten to fourteen days. If SE is less than 90% (85% for older adults), continue.

2. Limit your time in bed to your average TST, but not less than five hours. To accomplish this, set a consistent bedtime and rising time.

3. No daytime naps.

4. Adjust your time in bed:

   - When your average SE over a one-week period is 90% or more (85% for older adults), add fifteen minutes to your TIB.

   - If your one-week average SE is under 85% (80% for older adults), decrease your TIB to your current average TST, but not less than five hours.

   - If your SE is 85%–89% (80%–84% for older adults), make no change.

5. Repeat step 4 until you reach your target amount of sleep.

6. Continue to log your sleep each night.

Sleep Restriction Therapy: Detailed Instructions

Now let's look closely at each step. Though the steps may seem simple in concept, clients usually have quite a few questions once they start to think about actually doing the program.

1. Calculate your average total sleep time (TST), average time in bed (TIB), and sleep efficiency (SE) using sleep log data for ten to fourteen days. If SE is less than 90% (85% for older adults), continue.

Your sleep efficiency is the proportion of time in bed that you are asleep. Most people do spend some time (ten to twenty minutes) awake before dropping off to sleep in the beginning of the night. It also is completely normal to have one or two brief awakenings (depending on your age and other factors). Thus, we don't expect 100% efficiency. A good target is 90% for youth and adults, and 85% for older adults, since people do have more awakenings with age (Williams, Karacan & Hursch, 1974).

There are times to use SRT even if your average SE is over 90%. For example, if your SE was high only on nights you used sleep aids, this will pull up your average. You can calculate your average total sleep time using only the nights on which you did not use sleep aids. This then forms the basis for your initial SRT prescription. Also, if your technical SE is over 90% because you do not stay in bed when you are not asleep, but you are asleep less than 90% of the time between your initial bedtime and final rise time, SRT can certainly work well.

2. Limit your time in bed to your average TST, but not less than five hours. To accomplish this, set a consistent bedtime and rising time.

Remember, it is best to use ten to fourteen nights of sleep log data to determine your current average TST. If you are currently averaging over five hours of sleep, you will set your TIB equal to your average TST. Otherwise, you will set your TIB to five hours. The developers of this treatment started with a lower limit of four hours and thirty minutes prescribed TIB, but increased this to five hours because less than five hours was creating too much sleep deprivation in the beginning of treatment, without enough added benefit to outweigh this cost (Spielman, Chien-Ming & Glovinsky, 2011).

Once you figure out how many hours you will be in bed, how do you choose *which* hours? There are different philosophies about this. We tend to share the view of the people who developed SRT: we suggest setting your sleep window during the stretch of night that is most likely to contain your best sleep (Spielman, Chien-Ming & Glovinsky, 2011). For example, if you fall asleep easily and get several hours of solid sleep before waking up, start your sleep window at your desired bedtime. If, on the other hand, the early part of the night is hardest, and you finally drop into a deep sleep at 3 a.m., then set your sleep window for the latter part of the night, waking up at your desired rise time. If it is the middle stretch that brings the most tranquil sleep, shave off time in bed at both ends. If there is no predictable pattern or your sleep is equally fitful throughout the night, consider what schedule will be easiest for you. Is it easier to imagine staying up later, or getting out of bed earlier?

If, after considering all of this, you still are not sure, our default is to have you go to bed later and rise at your desired wake time. We say this because (1) a majority of our clients say that it is easier to force themselves to stay awake later than it is to force themselves out of bed before sunrise; and (2) having a fixed wake time is one of the best anchors for your internal clock, and you will not have to adjust your wake time during the treatment program if you start with it at your desired rise time.

By "desired bedtime" we mean the time you hope to go to bed once your sleep has regulated. If you would normally shoot for 10:30 p.m.–6 a.m., but have been getting in bed at 9 p.m. because you're so exhausted, start your sleep window no earlier than 10:30 p.m. By "desired rise time," we do not mean in your ideal world, but rather the earliest you have to be up to meet your obligations (child care, work, school) or participate in desired activities (worship services, running group). So if twice a week you need to be up by 6:30, have your rise time be no later than 6:30. Having a consistent sleep-wake schedule—not just a restricted one—is an essential component of SRT.

3. No daytime naps.

Even short naps will lower your sleep drive. We are not sure, but even tiny "nod offs" close to bed may make a big difference in some people's sleep drive. A stronger sleep drive will help you fall asleep quickly and stay asleep throughout the night.

4. Adjust your time in bed: When your average SE over a one-week period is 90% (85% for older adults) or more, add fifteen minutes to your TIB. If your one-week average SE is under 85% (80% for older adults), decrease your TIB to your current average TST, but not less than five hours. If your SE is 85%–89% (80%–84% for older adults), make no change.

It is essential that you continue to keep your sleep log as you do SRT. Not only will this help you honestly evaluate how closely you are sticking with the program, it also will provide the information you need to know when it is time to increase (or decrease) your time in bed. Notice in this instruction that you are changing your TIB based on a full week of data, not just one night. This (1) allows you to build the solid base of consolidated sleep we are seeking, (2) protects against "kneejerk" reactions to one unusually "good" or "bad" night, and (3) may keep you from putting too much pressure on yourself to sleep on any one particular night.

By a "one-week period" we mean any consecutive seven days, not necessarily a calendar week. You are welcome to calculate your averages just once a week, or you can do it more frequently using the previous seven nights' data. For example, say your SE is 88% in the first week of treatment (leading you to keep your TIB the same), and was clearly better the last four nights than the first three. Instead of waiting another seven nights, you may want to see if your SE has reached the 90% threshold after three more days on the program. If your seven-day average SE is now 90%, you can increase your TIB after ten nights, instead of waiting a full two weeks.

Very rarely do our clients have to reduce their TIB *if* their initial prescription was set at their current average TST. It is theoretically possible that your sleep will become even less efficient during the program, and your SE will fall in the range that suggests you decrease TIB. However, we have only had this happen with clients who started with a more gentle restriction, and therefore could not really expect to sleep 85% of the time they were in bed.

5. Repeat step 4 until you reach your target amount of sleep.

Think of your target as the amount of sleep that allows you to feel rested and perform well during the day. There is no one ideal for everyone. In fact, your own sleep needs are likely to change over time.

You may discover through this program that you need less sleep than you thought. For example, right now you may think that you do best with eight hours. Let's say in the first six weeks of treatment you are hitting the 90% SE mark and you add fifteen minutes TIB each week. Now, in week 7, you increase TIB to seven and a half hours and your sleep breaks apart some, yielding an SE of less than 85%. You decide to return to seven and a quarter hours TIB, and realize that you are feeling rested and there are no negative daytime consequences. We would celebrate this as a success. The goal of treatment is not to get to some predetermined amount of sleep that you *think* you need, but to get the sleep that you actually do need. We want to help you sleep to live, not live to sleep. Focusing on how you feel during the day—instead of how much sleep you are getting at night—is a big part of this.

Common Questions (and Answers) or Roadblocks (and Possible Solutions)

"You want me to RESTRICT my sleep, when I'm already getting too little? No way!"

We cannot tell you how many times we have witnessed people convert from "no way" to true believers. This treatment works! It may help to realize that although the treatment is called *sleep* restriction, we are restricting your *time in bed* more than your actual sleep. A better, less alarming name might be "sleep consolidation therapy."

Realistically, though, you probably will get less sleep at first. You will be in bed for the amount of time you currently are sleeping, and we expect you to sleep about 90% of the time you are in bed, which means you may get 10% less sleep than your current average. For example, if you are averaging six hours of TST, you will get closer to five and a half hours of sleep if your SE is 90%. Now, if you follow the program strictly, you may be so tired that your SE is well over 90% and you may not lose sleep. Also, even if you get less sleep, your sleep may quickly become deeper and more restorative, leading you to feel better instead of worse. Even if you do feel worse at first, we are confident that this will pay off in the long term.

Some clinicians do suggest an initial prescription of thirty minutes more than your average TST. This extra padding makes it more likely that you will not initially lose sleep, making the program more palatable or acceptable to some people. You can certainly try this more lenient approach. We suggest the more aggressive approach because we have seen this work better for more people.

"Can I do a more mild version of the treatment?"

Perhaps you are currently sleeping an average of six hours a night, are in bed nine hours, and want to know if you can limit TIB to seven hours instead of six. Remember, you do not "have" to do anything we suggest! In our experience, a smaller "dose" of the treatment does sometimes work. And sometimes it doesn't. Ask yourself: do you prefer to be aggressive, so that you are more likely to get quicker results? Or do you prefer to be a bit more gentle, perhaps to have less anxiety about the treatment or to feel more confident that you can handle your daytime obligations?

Most of our clients who start with a more gentle prescription end up reducing their TIB more before they get the results they are looking for. Interestingly, there is a treatment called "sleep compression" that has you gradually decrease your TIB until it matches your

TST. In the example above, you would start by restricting TIB to seven and a half hours, which is halfway between your average TST and TIB. The following week you would reduce to six and three-quarters hours, and then the next week to six hours. We suggest SRT instead of sleep compression if you are willing to be more aggressive, because it works more quickly.

"My baseline sleep logs show an average TST of four hours. Can I restrict my TIB below five hours, to be even more aggressive?"

We suggest that you start with five hours of TIB. If you do not make significant progress and are safely tolerating the sleep deprivation, then you may decide to restrict your TIB further. If you are going to restrict TIB below five hours, we recommend that you be in bed for at least thirty minutes more than your current TST since you are unlikely to sleep the entire time you are in bed, and you are getting so little sleep already. In this example, then, you would set TIB to four and a half hours.

"Once in a while I have to get up earlier than usual, but I really don't want this to be my regular rise time. What should I do?"

Although having a consistent sleep-wake schedule is important, remember our emphasis on finding the sweet spot: be as consistent as you can be so the program has the best chance of working, but flexible enough to tailor the program to your own needs. Let's say you usually need to rise at 7 a.m. but once every two weeks you have to be up at 6:15. If 7 a.m. is a much more appealing rise time, you may decide to have an inconsistent sleep schedule once every two weeks, rather than an undesirable rise time every morning.

"My prescribed sleep window starts really late. What should I do until bedtime?"

Whatever you want! You can stay out later socializing, reading at a coffee shop, or grocery shopping. You can get house chores or work done. You can engage in your favorite hobbies. You can do something indulgent that you ordinarily don't take the time to do. We do suggest a wind-down period (see chapter 9). It is just that this buffer between your day and your sleep may be at 1 a.m. instead of 10 p.m.

Some people do struggle to stay awake. You may feel too tired to safely be out of your home, and may not have the energy or focus for chores, work, or your hobbies. You may doze off with a less demanding activity like watching television. First, consider recruiting someone to spend time with you (even if by telephone). Do you have any "night owls" in your life, or people who live in a different time zone so that they will be awake when you are struggling? Do you have a housemate who would be happy to stay up late with you? Second, spend some time brainstorming activities that are possible with your level of energy, provide enough stimulation to keep you awake, and won't disturb others in your household. This is different for everyone. Maybe reading feels impossible, but you can listen to an audio book. Maybe you are too unfocused to manage your finances, but you can sort and file papers that have been screaming for organization. Other ideas from some of our clients: prepare tomorrow's meals; fold or iron laundry; clean or organize; play games like Sudoku or solitaire; organize photographs; write (letters, stories, journals); stretch or do a nighttime yoga routine; take a bath; watch television or movies; plan an upcoming vacation; or do crafts like knitting, sewing, scrapbooking, or wood whittling.

We do encourage you to make these hours rewarding. The last thing we want is for you to view this treatment program as extending the hours of drudgery in each day. If all the time you have been spending trying to sleep has gotten you behind, and you are getting more and more overwhelmed with life's chores, then maybe it will be more rewarding to get stuff done. On the other hand, if you have been pushing through everything you "have to" or "should" do, with little time or energy left for simple pleasures, then we suggest that you do something more relaxing or indulgent.

"My prescribed sleep window suggests that I get up really early. I'm afraid I won't be able to."

This can take some significant problem-solving, and the solutions available depend on your living environment. If you have a housemate who rises early, see if he or she will help you. We have had some clients whose spouse or parents woke them with a cup of coffee in hand! Or perhaps someone not in the house would be willing to call you. Or maybe, based on the guidelines above, you initially set your sleep window to a 4 a.m. wakeup and your bed partner rises at 4:45. You may decide to set your rise time in sync with your partner's in order to make it easier for you to comply.

If you need to depend on an alarm but sleep through even the loudest, you may benefit from a bed-shaking alarm or a timer that turns on your lights. If you are prone to turning off the alarm and falling promptly back to sleep, you may need multiple alarms, including one or more that is out of reach of the bed. There are alarm clocks that move around the room so that you have to chase after them. There are smartphone applications that make you do an alerting task—like swipe a particular pattern or scan a medication bottle—to turn off the alarm. We had a client set multiple alarms in a path from bed to bathroom. Once in the bathroom, he got in the shower to keep from getting back in bed. Other clients put something on the bed to create an obstacle to climbing back in—one dumped a basket of laundry, while another scattered some marbles (ouch!).

"My prescribed sleep window suggests I get up really early. What should I do in the wee hours of the morning?"

On the one hand, we do not want you to train your brain to expect to start your day so early if your ultimate goal is to sleep later. On the other hand, we want you to recapture some of the time you have lost to insomnia, and we want you to experience these early morning hours as rewarding so that it is easier to stick with the program.

You may decide to simply start your day earlier, doing precisely what you would have done in the first hour after a more traditional wake time. Or you may decide to use these hours for pleasurable or self-care activities, such as exercise, reading, or watching movies. Or perhaps you want to get caught up on household tasks like cleaning or finances. Most of the information we provided above about what to do late at night applies here. Do you have a friend or relative who is a "morning lark" and would be interested in meeting for a walk or an early breakfast? Is there an exercise class you are interested in? It's amazing how much of the world is awake even at 5 a.m.!

If your ultimate goal is to be sleeping later, be careful not to make any long-term commitments that will not fit with your desired sleep schedule. For example, it is fine to go to a 5:15 a.m. exercise class this week if your prescribed wake time is 4:30. However, do not prepay for a three-month class at 5:15 a.m. if you hope to sleep until 6 a.m. later in the program.

"If I follow this program, I won't be going to bed with my bed partner. This is upsetting to me and/or to him or her."

First, if it is your partner you are worried about, check with him or her before you jump to conclusions. Explain what you are planning to do, why, and the fact that this will likely be a short-term change. (We say "likely" because your natural rhythm may be different than your partner's. Trying to go to sleep too early or too late may be part of your problem. If so, you may maintain a different sleep schedule even after the program.) We have been surprised how often our clients have expected their partners to be hurt or angry when they turned out to be supportive.

If you do not want to miss out on the connection you and your partner have at bedtime, you can climb in bed with your partner and then get out of bed when he or she falls asleep. This has worked really well for a couple of our clients!

"What's wrong with napping? Entire cultures revolve around a midday siesta!"

We are not asking you to give up naps forever. This program relies on your having a strong and consistent sleep drive at bedtime each night. Daytime naps will lower your sleep drive.

"My SE is over 90%. Can't I increase my TIB by more than a piddly fifteen minutes?"

You can, but we generally do not recommend it. The developers of the treatment suggest increasing TIB in fifteen- or thirty-minute increments (Spielman, Chien-Ming & Glovinsky, 2011). We suggest fifteen minutes because when our clients have tried to take bigger steps, more often than not their sleep has broken apart more. Sometimes it was then hard for them to recapture their initial improvements.

"Can't I increase my TIB more frequently if my SE is high?"

Again, you can, but we do not recommend it. There is nothing magical about seven nights, so we can't argue that you should absolutely wait seven instead of adjusting after five nights, for example. And there are not any research studies comparing different versions of SRT. But just like with the amount of time you add at each step, our experience suggests that "the slower you go, the faster you get there."

Our experience also supports flexibility. If there is a compelling reason to increase your TIB after five or six nights, we would certainly support you in trying this.

"My average SE for the past week is 90%, but the past two nights haven't been so great. Should I increase my TIB tonight?"

If you are willing to be patient and take it slow, we recommend continuing with your current TIB until your sleep is again more consolidated. You need not wait another week. If you sleep more solidly tonight, you may decide to increase TIB as soon as tomorrow night given your high weekly average SE.

"I set my sleep window to the part of the night when I sleep best, as you suggested. I am sleeping well during that time, but I can't seem to sleep more now that I've increased my TIB."

Remember how we said that there are different philosophies? You may want to use the competing philosophy: schedule your sleep window for the part of the night that contains your worst or least reliable sleep. The hope is that this will force you to sleep during the most difficult hours. It will then be easier to expand your sleep into the part of the night that contains your best sleep.

For example, if you sleep well in the beginning of the night, you will now stay awake during these hours. When you finally go to sleep for the last part of your target sleep window, your sleep drive will be so high that you will be more likely to sleep. When it is time to increase your TIB, you will do so by going to bed earlier. This likely will not be a problem because you will be going to bed at a time of night when you tend to sleep better.

"I'm fighting off a cold or flu. What should I do?"

Our bodies do need more rest when we are sick or getting sick. If you are actually able to sleep deeply, you may decide to suspend treatment and let your body get the sleep it needs. However, if you are resting more than you are sleeping, or if your sleep is fitful or broken, we encourage you to give your body the rest it needs while keeping the SRT principles in place. That is, outside of your prescribed sleep window, rest on a couch or chair, preferably without nodding off. Rest in bed during your prescribed window.

"I want to start SRT now, but I'm in the middle of tapering off of a benzodiazepine. What do I need to know?"

We have had plenty of clients do SRT at the same time they are coming off of a benzodiazepine medication (generally prescribed for sleep or anxiety) because they are tapering very slowly and do not want to delay SRT for weeks or months. The main thing to avoid is changing your medication dose and your TIB at the same time. We generally recommend five days between changes (though this is not based on research because we are unaware of any data on this). For example, if your SE is 90%, but you just decreased your medication dose, hold steady your TIB for another five nights. Then add fifteen minutes, but only if your SE is still 90% or more. Similarly, if you just increased your TIB, wait at least five nights before decreasing your medication dose.

The idea is to let your body adjust to the change you just made (decreased medication or increased TIB) before introducing another change. If this advice is counter to a schedule your physician gave you for coming off of your medications, please consult with your physician.

"I'm going to be traveling across time zones. How should I handle this?"

If it works to keep your sleep window the same based on your home time zone, this is least disruptive and we would default to this. However, you may need to be awake at different hours (if, for example, you are traveling east and have early morning commitments). There is not one right way to shift your sleep window. We mostly want you to think it through ahead of time, and pick a plan in which you have confidence. Some people slowly shift their sleep window before they travel. Others slowly shift it once they arrive at their destination. Others shift all at once instead of slowly. And some shift their sleep window to hours somewhere between their home and travel time zones.

"Daylight Savings Time is starting (or ending). How should I handle this?"

The same principles apply here as with travel. If you don't need to adjust your hours, don't. If you do need to, you can do it all at once, or incrementally. Let's say your target sleep window is 10 p.m.–6 a.m. If your current sleep window is 11 p.m.–4 a.m., then you can continue to sleep at the same "sun time" when the clocks change. Shifting one hour in either direction keeps you in your target range. Similarly, you can stay on the same sleep schedule if your current sleep window is 1 a.m.–6 a.m. and the clocks are moving back, though the clock will now read 12 midnight to 5 a.m. If you do this, then you will need to add TIB to both ends of the sleep window over the course of treatment, rather than just moving your bedtime earlier.

If, however, your current sleep window is 1 a.m.–6 a.m., and the clocks are moving forward, then you will need to adjust your sleep window in order to stay within your target sleep window. On the Saturday night of the time change, you can go to bed and get up an hour earlier *if* you have been very sleepy in the hour before your current bedtime and are confident that you will fall asleep easily. Otherwise, you may want to shift your sleep window earlier in increments of fifteen to thirty minutes. (You can also use some of your extra time out of bed to lobby your congressional representatives to do away with Daylight Savings Time!)

"I just don't want to [spend less time in bed, give up even more sleep]!"

You don't have to *want* to do a particular thing in order to do it. Try this: think of all the things you have done even though you did not want to. Have you paid taxes or bills that you did not want to pay? Waited in a line when you would have liked to walk right up to the register? Sat squished in the middle seat on an airplane? Scrubbed a toilet or done other housework that you hate doing? Attended a family function you wanted to skip? Completed a class you did not like? Chances are you have done thousands of things that you have not wanted to do.

Sometimes when we want to get somewhere, we do not enjoy every part of the journey. This may be true of your journey to better sleep. If you do not want to do this treatment fully, we urge you to take a few moments to think about your goals. Why are you reading this book? What do you want to change? How might your life be better if SRT works for you? Now, carefully consider: are you willing to spend less time in bed—and possibly sleep a little less—in the service of these goals?

If you simply are not willing to follow the SRT guidelines, then you can consider stimulus control. If this is not an option (based on your work in chapter 5, or because you are not willing to do that either), then you can start with cognitive strategies, especially working with the thoughts that are interfering with your willingness to do the behavioral programs.

"I have bipolar disorder [or a seizure disorder]. Are you sure I can't do this program?"

No! We have had success using SRT with clients who have bipolar disorder or other conditions that are sensitive to decreased sleep. However, because of the increased risk of negative consequences (such as increased mood instability), we strongly suggest that you work with a knowledgeable clinician who can help you decide whether and when to use the program, modify the program as needed, and monitor your symptoms.

What to Expect

You may be wondering how long it will take for this treatment to work. Your sleep may improve almost immediately: by giving yourself less time in bed, your sleep may quickly consolidate, leading you to feel more rested even with less sleep. Or, even if your sleep isn't more refreshing, you may feel a lot better because you have recaptured hours of your life that you had given over to insomnia. One client came in after the first week of SRT amazed at how good it felt to go to his office. In response to his insomnia he had been working from home so that he could cater to his erratic sleep schedule and take breaks when he needed to. He hadn't realized how isolated he felt, nor how guilty he felt about "taking advantage" of a flexible manager. With his SRT prescription, he knew he had to be out of bed for many more hours, and decided that it would actually be easier to stick to the program if he was at the office instead of near a bed. As his daytime quality of life improved, so too did his ability to sleep at night.

Many people, though, feel worse before they feel better. As acknowledged above, you may get about 10% less sleep than your pretreatment average since you are unlikely to sleep 100% of the time that you are in bed. And if you have some nights that are better than others, you will be giving up the extra sleep you were getting on the best nights by restricting yourself to only an average night's sleep. Plus, if you feel anxious about restricting your sleep window, anxious arousal may make you sleep worse than usual.

If you do feel worse at first, please know that this does not mean that the treatment isn't working! In fact, this may even work in your favor. Lost sleep tonight can ramp up your sleep drive, improving your sleep on subsequent nights. If you stick with SRT, we have very high confidence that the program will work, and you will soon be feeling better.

Finally, at some point during the program you may feel more groggy when you wake up, and you may conclude that you are even more sleep deprived than before. Believe it or not, this can be an encouraging sign: we feel more groggy when we are pulled out of deeper stages of sleep, so your grogginess may mean you are getting more deep sleep, which is exactly what we are hoping for!

You may be worn down from months or years or even decades of insomnia. We know that this can make it incredibly hard to risk getting even less sleep or feeling even more tired. We would not ask you to do this hard work if we had not witnessed the dramatic improvements our clients have had using this treatment. Nor would we ask you to do this hard work if we knew of an easier and more comfortable way.

Whether you improve quickly or it takes weeks, your improvement may not be linear. You may make progress and then suffer a setback. Most often a setback will come when you have just increased your TIB. With time, your sleep is likely to consolidate again. If it does not consolidate during the week, and your SE has dipped below the 85% threshold, you will decrease your TIB. We know this can be discouraging, but don't give up! If you stick with the program, it is likely to work. Sometimes our bodies need to hang out at a new plateau before more change is possible. Weight loss is a good example. If you want to lose twenty pounds and you change your eating and exercise habits to accomplish this, the first five pounds may come off quickly. Then the scale may stop moving. If you are accepting of this and are willing to stay at this weight while you continue to eat and exercise for weight loss, your body will eventually adjust to its new weight and you will again start to lose. If, on the other hand, you become discouraged and return to your old eating and exercise habits, you will regain the five pounds (and maybe more). Similarly, if you were getting an average of five hours of sleep before this program and now the needle is stuck at six, we encourage you to keep with the program. Six reliable hours of sleep at the same time each night really is a significant improvement, and we are confident you can build on this, even if it is going slower than you would like.

How long can you expect to be doing the SRT program? You can calculate the shortest amount of time it will take you to reach your target: take the difference between your goal TST and your starting prescribed TST, and divide by 15 if you are using minutes, or multiply by 4 if you are using hours; this is the number of weeks the treatment will take if you are able to increase TIB by 15 minutes each week. For example: if you desire 7½ hours of sleep and start with 5¾ hours in bed, the difference is 105 minutes (or 1.75 hours). 105/15 = 7 (or 1.75 × 4 = 7), so the program will take at least seven weeks to complete. In our experience people usually spend a little more time on the program.

However, if you are aggressive (starting with TIB equal to TST, and really sticking to the program each night) you likely will feel significantly better within three to five weeks of starting the program. The last few weeks on the program will be relatively easy because you will be getting consistent, predictable, good-quality sleep, which you haven't had in a long time. Plus, even though you will not yet be at your goal, you will be getting more sleep than before treatment. So do not get too discouraged when you calculate how long the program will take you. You likely will get significant relief in less time!

Your Sleep Restriction Therapy Plan

Use worksheet 7.1 to develop your personalized SRT plan. Really think about each part of the plan. (How will you stay awake? How will you wake up? Why are you willing to do this?) Ask yourself if you are willing to commit to the treatment plan you just devised. You do not have to know for how long you are willing to commit. It is enough to be fully committed today. You can recommit tomorrow.

WORKSHEET 7.1: Your Sleep Restriction Therapy Plan

Sleep Restriction Therapy: Basic Recipe

1. Calculate your average total sleep time (TST), average time in bed (TIB), and sleep efficiency (SE) using sleep log data for ten to fourteen days. If SE is less than 90% (85% for older adults), continue.

2. Limit your time in bed to your average TST, but not less than five hours. To accomplish this, set a consistent bedtime and rising time.

3. No daytime naps.

4. Adjust your time in bed:

   - When your average SE over a one-week period is 90% or more (85% for older adults), add fifteen minutes to your TIB.

   - If your one-week average SE is under 85% (80% for older adults), decrease your TIB to your current average TST, but not less than five hours.

   - If your SE is 85%–89% (80%–84% for older adults), make no change.

5. Repeat step 4 until you reach your target amount of sleep.

6. Continue to log your sleep each night.

My Prescription: My pretreatment average total sleep time = _____ hours.

Start Date	TIB (hrs)	Bedtime	Rise Time	Start Date	TIB (hrs)	Bedtime	Rise Time
1.				5.			
2.				6.			
3.				7.			
4.				8.			

Strategies for staying awake until my prescribed bedtime:

Strategies for getting up at my prescribed wake time:

Activities I can do in the extra time I'm spending out of bed:

What I will have to give up (for example, "sleeping in on weekends," "falling asleep for one last stretch right around my wake time"):

What discomfort I may experience (for example, "I may be even more tired at first," "loneliness being up alone late at night or early in the morning"):

Why I'm willing to give these things up (for now) and experience these discomforts (for now):

Your Next Step

Once you have started your SRT program, you can start to work on other strategies that are part of your treatment plan (refer to worksheet 5.1). However, be sure to stay focused on your SRT program. Remember, SRT and SCT are really the backbone of CBT-I and we would rather you do one treatment component fully than do several parts of the treatments in watered-down fashion.

Continue to track your sleep with the sleep log. Be as accurate and honest as you can be about what time you got into bed and what time you got out. This will help you evaluate how closely you are following the program. To help you decide when to change your TIB, you need to calculate your average total sleep time, time in bed, and sleep efficiency at the end of each week. Also record your weekly averages on your Sleep Log Summary (worksheet 5.2 or 5.3), and use this worksheet to track when you start SRT and other parts of your treatment program.

How to Evaluate Your Progress and When to Consider a Different Plan

In chapter 13 we will help you thoroughly evaluate your treatment program after six or eight weeks. But you also will be tracking your progress each week by calculating your sleep efficiency. What should you do if you are not sleeping for 90% of your sleep window?

First, look closely at your logs and at the SRT instructions and ask yourself how closely you are following the program. Did you start with a longer sleep window than your average TST? If so, are you willing and able to reduce your TIB to be more aggressive with the treatment? Or did you increase TIB before your SE reached 90%? Did you fail to decrease your TIB, even though your SE was under 85% and your TIB was over five hours? Finally, how closely are you sticking to your current TIB? Are you nodding off earlier than your bedtime, or sleeping through the alarm, or choosing to "sleep in, just this once"?

We have been surprised how often people say they did the treatment when their sleep logs show that they did not follow the guidelines very closely. If there is any room at all for improvement, the first thing we recommend is that you do the program even more fully. Are you willing to recommit to this treatment program? What would help you do so? If it is hard to do on your own, you may want to seek out a professional trained in CBT-I.

If you are doing the program fully and have had some clear improvement (you were able to add some TIB and your sleep is more consolidated) but have stalled out, we encourage you to continue. Remember, your body may need to hang out at a new plateau before it makes even more improvement.

If you have been doing the program fully for at least four weeks and are not improving at all, it may be time to switch to or add stimulus control.

Ready to set off on this leg of your adventure? Good luck!

Chapter 8

Combining Stimulus Control and Sleep Restriction

Stimulus control and sleep restriction are well-proven strategies to treat chronic insomnia, and they are thought to work by slightly different mechanisms. Stimulus control therapy (SCT) retrains your brain to more strongly associate bed with sleep (Bootzin & Perlis, 2011). Sleep restriction therapy (SRT) consolidates your sleep, making it less fragmented and more restorative, by giving your brain a shorter sleep window (Spielman, Chien-Ming & Glovinsky, 2011). It stands to reason that combining these two approaches will pack an even more powerful punch, as you simultaneously retrain your brain and consolidate your sleep.

Another reason to combine SCT and SRT is that there is some significant overlap in these two treatments. When you do SRT, you are in bed less and you are asleep for more of the time that you are in bed. This is right in line with the goal of SCT! Similarly, when you do SCT, you restrict your time in bed because you leave the bed when you are not sleeping. So these two treatments really complement each other.

Who Should Use Combined SCT-SRT?

Unfortunately, we are not aware of any research studies comparing SCT, SRT, and their combination. Therefore, we do not really know if the combination is more likely to give you better or quicker results. However, based on our experience, we encourage you to use the combined approach if you are:

- able to use the combined approach, and

- willing to do it fully.

By "able" we mean that exercise 5.2 led you to conclude that both SCT and SRT are safe for you, and both are possible with your sleep pattern. You already know what we mean by "willing to do it fully"! We do not suggest that you do two watered-down treatments. If you start with combined SCT-SRT and then feel that you have taken on too much, then choose either SCT or SRT and do it fully instead.

Why do we suggest the combined approach if you are willing and able to use it? In our experience, SRT often works more quickly than SCT. We often think of it as more powerful. However, SCT gives you a tool to use in the future, when you have just an occasional night of poor sleep. Imagine that treatment has gone well and you are getting fairly reliable, consolidated sleep. Then one night you have trouble falling asleep. What should you do? With SRT, there is no clear way to respond. Your sleep efficiency over the course of the week is still high, so restricting your time in bed is not necessary. It is perfectly okay to not respond to one lone night of disrupted sleep, if you can practice acceptance and not trigger an insomnia spiral. However, people who use SCT tell us that they love knowing what to do when they cannot sleep. They say that it works better for them to get out of bed than to toss and turn and allow frustration or worry to build. So combining SCT and SRT may give you the best of both worlds: a quicker response, and a tool to maintain it!

Combined SCT and SRT: Basic Recipe

1. Limit your behavior in bed and in your bedroom to sleep and sex.

2. Calculate your average total sleep time (TST), average time in bed (TIB), and sleep efficiency (SE) using sleep log data for ten to fourteen days.

3. Limit your time in bed to your average TST, but not less than five hours. To accomplish this, set a consistent bedtime and rising time.

4. If, at any time during the night, you are awake for more than twenty minutes, leave the bedroom and do something boring or relaxing.

5. Return to bed when you are sleepy. (Do not sleep in another room.)

6. Repeat steps 4–5 as needed throughout the night.

7. Get up at your scheduled rising time regardless of how much sleep you got or how much time you spent in bed.

8. No daytime naps.

9. Continue to log your sleep each night.

10. Adjust your time in bed:

    *   When you are sleeping an average of 90% or more (85% for older adults) of your sleep window over a one-week period, add fifteen minutes to your TIB.

    *   If your one-week average SE is under 85% (80% for older adults), decrease your TIB to your current average TST, but not less than five hours.

    *   If your SE is 85%–89% (80%–84% for older adults), make no change.

11. Repeat step 10 until you reach your target amount of sleep.

Combined SCT-SRT: Detailed Instructions

As you can see, in this combined SCT-SRT program you limit your sleep window to the number of hours you are currently sleeping, *and* you leave your bedroom if you are awake for more than twenty minutes. Let's say you currently get six hours of sleep on average, and you pick a sleep schedule of 12 midnight to 6 a.m. Before midnight, you will be out of your room as much as possible, using it only to prepare for bed or put laundry away, for example. You will climb into bed at midnight and give yourself up to twenty minutes to fall asleep. You will also give yourself up to twenty minutes to fall back to sleep if you wake in the middle of the night. If, at any point, you are awake for longer than twenty minutes, or if you become anxious or frustrated, you will leave the bedroom and go to a predetermined place and do something that is boring or relaxing. You will return to bed when you are sleepy. You will once again leave your bed if you are not asleep within twenty minutes. Regardless of how much or how little you have slept, you will get out of bed at 6 a.m. and will, once again, spend as little waking time as possible in your bedroom. You will not nap during the day. As your sleep knits together and you start to sleep an average of 90% of your sleep window, you will add fifteen minutes to your time in bed, up to once per week.

Notice that in this program we suggest you calculate sleep efficiency (SE) using your *sleep window* rather than your actual time in bed, which will be different if you get out of bed during your sleep window because of the stimulus control part of the treatment. Think of your sleep window as the time between lights out and your final rise time. In the example above, if you stick to your prescription and go to bed at midnight and get out of bed for the final time at 6 a.m. each day, then your average sleep window will be six hours. If you cannot sleep and you get up and read for an hour, you will still use six hours instead of using five hours of TIB to calculate your sleep efficiency that night. This is because we want you sleeping at least 90% of your prescribed *sleep window* before you increase your time in bed. If you are prescribed six hours, are out of bed for two hours, and sleep close to four hours, your SE calculated the traditional way will be over 90%, but it doesn't actually make sense to add time in bed when you are only sleeping for two-thirds of your prescribed time!

This different way of calculating your SE is really the only thing that is different from the instructions for doing either SCT and SRT alone. Rather than repeat all of these instructions here, we would like you to read chapters 6 and 7 (if you have not already done so) before starting a combined SCT-SRT program. In those chapters you will find detailed instructions for all of the steps in this combined approach (for example, what are some activities you can do if you cannot sleep and you leave your bed during your sleep window?

How should you choose your bedtime and rise time?). You will also find answers to the most common questions and challenges our clients bring to us.

Your Combined SCT-SRT Plan

Now that you have reviewed chapters 6 and 7, complete worksheet 8.1 to develop your personalized combined SCT-SRT program. Take your time and carefully consider each part of the plan. (How will you keep yourself awake for so long? Where will you go and what will you do if you cannot sleep during your sleep window?) If you need to make any preparations—such as gathering reading material or asking someone to help you get up at your rise time—do this ahead of time.

Before you start, check in with yourself. How willing are you to start this program? Can you fully commit to the plan you just developed? If you can commit to it tonight, that is enough. You can commit again tomorrow, and the day after, and the day after that.

WORKSHEET 8.1: Your Combined Stimulus Control Therapy and Sleep Restriction Therapy Plan

Combined SCT and SRT: Basic Recipe

1. Limit your behavior in bed and in your bedroom to sleep and sex.

2. Calculate your average total sleep time (TST), average time in bed (TIB), and sleep efficiency (SE) using sleep log data for ten to fourteen days.

3. Limit your time in bed to your average TST, but not less than five hours. To accomplish this, set a consistent bedtime and rising time.

4. If, at any time during the night, you are awake for more than twenty minutes, leave the bedroom and do something boring or relaxing.

5. Return to bed when you are sleepy. (Do not sleep in another room.)

6. Repeat steps 4–5 as needed throughout the night.

7. Get up at your scheduled rising time regardless of how much sleep you got or how much time you spent in bed.

8. No daytime naps.

9. Continue to log your sleep each night.

10. Adjust your time in bed:

    - When you are sleeping an average of 90% or more (85% for older adults) of your sleep window over a one-week period, add fifteen minutes to your TIB.

    - If your one-week average SE is under 85% (80% for older adults), decrease your TIB to your current average TST, but not less than five hours.

    - If your SE is 85%–89% (80%–84% for older adults), make no change.

11. Repeat step 10 until you reach your target amount of sleep.

My Prescription: My pretreatment average total sleep time = _____ hours.

Start Date	TIB (hrs)	Bedtime	Rise Time	Start Date	TIB (hrs)	Bedtime	Rise Time
1.				5.			
2.				6.			
3.				7.			
4.				8.			

Strategies for staying awake until my prescribed bedtime:

Strategies for getting up at my prescribed wake time:

Activities I can do in the extra time I'm spending out of bed:

If I leave my bed because I'm not sleeping during my sleep window...

This is where in my home I will go:

These are activities I will engage in (*be specific!*):

Preparations to make ahead of time (for example, set multiple alarms, put low-watt bulb in lamp):

Strategies for avoiding naps or nodding off:

What I will have to give up (for example, "sleeping in on weekends," "falling asleep for one last stretch right around my wake time," "the comfort of going to sleep to the TV"):

What discomfort I may experience (for example, "I may be even more tired at first," "Loneliness being up alone late at night or early in the morning," "Guilt for disturbing my partner"):

Why I'm willing to give these things up (for now) and experience these discomforts (for now):

Your Next Step

Once your combined SCT-SRT program is under way, you are welcome to start working on sleep hygiene or the cognitive strategies that are part of your personalized treatment plan (worksheet 5.1).

Make sure you continue to track your sleep with the sleep log. Mark when you get into and out of bed (in the beginning, middle, and end of the night). Each morning, estimate the total number of hours you slept. This will help you evaluate how closely you are following the program, and also will help you determine when you should increase (or decrease) the amount of time you spend in bed.

At the end of each week, calculate your averages and use your Sleep Log Summary form to help you track your sleep and your treatments. Use the information in the preceding two chapters and in chapter 13 to help you decide what to do if your sleep is not improving.

You have taken on an ambitious treatment program. If you do it fully, you may be really tired at first, but there is an excellent chance that your sleep will improve and you will soon feel much better. Good luck!

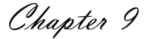

Chapter 9

Sleep Hygiene

Yyou may remember from chapter 2 that your internal body clock and your sleep drive are your body's two big players in healthy sleep, and they are both impacted by what you do. Sleep hygiene guidelines are largely focused on what you can do—or refrain from doing—to positively impact your body clock and its synchronicity with the sleep drive. Sleep hygiene also includes guidelines for creating optimal conditions for a sleep-promoting environment, such as a comfortable bed and room. The questions about sleep hygiene practices that you answered in chapter 5 should have illuminated which guidelines you follow closely and which may be targets for change. We encourage you to assess your sleep hygiene from the perspective of "What am I currently doing to *support* my sleep?" and from that of "What am I currently doing that may *disrupt* my sleep?" Considering both perspectives can be helpful in uncovering well-intentioned but sleep-disruptive behaviors.

Sleep hygiene is analogous to oral hygiene practices—such as flossing, brushing, and minimizing sugary foods—that support healthy teeth and gums. You can do a great job with oral hygiene and still get a cavity. When you go to the dentist, you expect the dentist to tell you to keep flossing and brushing, but you do not expect the dentist to tell you that the cavity will be fixed by continued or improved oral hygiene. The cavity is a separate issue that requires additional intervention. Chronic insomnia and other sleep problems are the same. You will want to engage in effective sleep hygiene, but your chronic sleep problems need additional components of CBT-I, such as stimulus control or sleep restriction.

It is interesting to note that people who have trouble sleeping typically also have a hard time with sleep hygiene and are more likely to engage in behaviors that disrupt sleep, such as napping or drinking alcohol before bedtime (Jefferson et al., 2005). Though there is no definitive answer as to why this is true, we have come to believe that poor sleepers are more reactive to sleep concerns, paying more attention to, and feeling a greater urgency to "fix," any sleep disruption they experience. Though well intentioned, these efforts to fix the problem or compensate for lack of sleep tend to be counter to sleep hygiene guidelines and actually create more problems. This notion supports our discussion in chapter 2 about the value of a paradigm shift: we invite you to take this opportunity to shift your focus from fixing or avoiding your immediate sleep issues, to promoting and optimizing your healthy sleep over the long term.

In this chapter we will review the most common sleep hygiene guidelines and help you assess your willingness to change your behaviors or sleep environment to be more consistent with these guidelines. Some of these changes will involve adding behaviors (such as establishing a bedtime routine) and others will involve removing behaviors (such as cutting out alcohol before bed). Either way, we are talking about change, and behavioral change can be challenging. Therefore, we also offer some general tips to help you succeed.

Sleep Hygiene Guidelines

Understanding the rationale behind any suggestion can help you make and maintain a behavioral change. This is why we believe it is so important to learn about sleep physiology—our understanding of the physiology of sleep provides the rationale for all of the behavioral programs in this book, including sleep hygiene. Therefore, as we review each sleep hygiene guideline, we also will explain why it is important. The core message is this: if you get out of your own way, your body will naturally self-correct, leading to reliable, restorative sleep.

Maintain a consistent sleep schedule.

A consistent schedule supports your body clock by giving it environmental cues, such as your first exposure to light, at the same time each day. An inconsistent schedule, on the other hand, confuses your body clock and makes your body work harder to maintain consistent wake and sleep cycles. A sleep schedule is important to your body clock not just this night but the next night and the next night as the body clock forms this rhythm over weeks and months.

It is most important that you have a consistent wake time. If you wake up at the same time regardless of what time you went to sleep the night before, this will help your body stay in rhythm. If you always get up at 7 a.m., for example, then your sleep drive will be at the same place at 11 p.m. each night, making it more likely that you will have a consistent bedtime when life does not interfere. We encourage you to stay within thirty to forty-five minutes of your target wake time, no matter how sleepy you are, even on weekends. Of course, during a stimulus control or sleep restriction program, you will have even less variability in your wake time.

A consistent bedtime is also useful, but you likely will have some variability here. For example, you may have an evening engagement that keeps you up later than usual; we do not want you to become a slave to sleep, and prefer that you enjoy meaningful activities even if this creates variability in your bedtime. Also, we generally suggest that you not go to sleep at your target bedtime if you are not sleepy, since this is a setup for lying in bed awake. Thus, we encourage you to establish a target bedtime, and to strive to maintain consistency, while accepting some variability. Remember, if you wake up at your normal time even after a late night, this will help your body stay in rhythm.

Have a brisk wakeup, and get natural light within one hour of waking.

It is helpful to make the transition from sleeping to waking as quickly as possible. You can liken this to pulling a Band-aid off your skin quickly; the faster you make the transition the faster you adjust and move through any discomfort. This means resisting the urge to hit the snooze button. It also means that it is better to get up than to doze in and out, even if you wake up before your desired wake time. It also helps if you get natural light within the first hour of waking. Light will cue your body clock to start your wake cycle for the day; for example, it will suppress your body's production of melatonin, a hormone that provides a cue for sleepiness. If you cannot get bright natural light at your wake time, consider using a light source that mimics the spectrum of natural daylight. We discuss these types of resources in appendix A (Circadian Rhythm Disorders).

Eliminate or limit napping.

Napping can confuse your body clock and weaken your sleep drive, leading to trouble falling asleep as well as trouble staying asleep. We have found that, for some people, even nodding off briefly seems to interfere with the body clock: brief snatches of sleep seem to signal to the brain that it is now time to be awake, even though you are far from rested. If you choose to nap, consider napping for no more than twenty to thirty minutes, and no later than midafternoon. If you tend to nod off before bed, we strongly encourage you to problem-solve to decrease the risk of this; for example, you may choose to sit on a more upright chair rather than reclining on a plush couch in the early evening, or you may walk briskly to the water fountain if your eyelids get heavy as you sit at your desk.

Eliminate or limit your stimulant intake.

Stimulants are any substance that activates your nervous system. Some typical stimulants are caffeine, sugar, and nicotine. If ingesting these, it is best to do so early in the day, before noon. Be conscious of both the obvious sources of caffeine, such as coffee, tea, soda, and energy drinks, and also less obvious sources such as medicines (for example, Excedrin, Midol, or decongestants) and smoothies with "energy boosts." Eliminating or reducing stimulants allows your body clock to follow its natural rhythms. Using stimulants impacts your body clock by increasing the amount of time your nervous system is activated, and may get your body clock out of sync with your sleep drive (look back at figure 2.1 for a better understanding of this).

Avoid activating medications at night.

We have already mentioned medications that contain caffeine, but even medications without caffeine can have an effect on your wake and sleep patterns. Perhaps the most common over-the-counter culprits are decongestants, which have an activating effect. We also have worked with people who were taking a stimulating antidepressant (such as Wellbutrin) or stimulant (such as Adderall or Ritalin) too late in the day. A medication that makes someone else sleepy may make you alert, and vice versa. Check the common side effects of your medications and consult your medical provider to determine if you can move potentially stimulating medications to earlier in the day, and more sedating medications to later in the day.

Limit your use of alcohol and do not drink within three hours of bedtime.

Although alcohol may help you fall asleep, it interferes with the structure of sleep because your body is busy digesting and processing the alcohol rather than restoring your body and brain. Also, because alcohol is a muscle relaxant, your airway may be more likely to soften, which is especially concerning if you have sleep apnea.

Go to bed neither too hungry nor too full.

Aim for going to bed with a balanced appetite. A bedtime snack can be helpful. Although we most commonly see recommendations for a high carbohydrate/low protein snack, some of our clients find that the reverse—high protein/low carbohydrate—helps them sleep through the night. Whether you snack or have a late meal, be careful not to go to bed too full; you want enough food in your small intestine to help your body relax into sleeping without having to work at heavy digestion. In addition, acid reflux can be caused or made worse by lying down right after eating, and acid reflux can disturb your sleep even if you are completely unaware that you have it.

Exercise regularly, but not right before bed.

Regular physical exercise is an important anchor for sleep. Exercise helps you to get rid of excess stress hormones such as adrenaline and cortisol which, in excess, can interfere with your body clock's ability to initiate and maintain sleep. Exercise also raises your internal body temperature, and timing exercise to coincide with your natural rise in body temperature can further support your body clock. For optimal support with sleep, exercise around four or five hours prior to your bedtime. If you exercise at a different time of day, consider some light movement (such as jumping jacks or stairs) four or five hours before bed to provide this core heat. It is recommended that you avoid exercise close to your bedtime so as to avoid a temperature spike that may interfere with your sleep.

Engage in a wind-down routine.

In contrast to our suggestion that you quickly transition from sleep with a brisk wakeup, it is crucial that you dedicate time to support the transition from wake to sleep. We often encounter people who expect too much of their brains: they think they should be able to go, go, go all day and evening, and then fall asleep at a moment's notice. Our brains need a more gentle slowing. A wind-down routine that lasts twenty to sixty minutes will support your body clock in cueing your body to sleep. We encourage you to choose activities that are calming and to do them in low light. Some examples include listening to soothing music, doing some gentle stretching, reading, or engaging in a quiet hobby such as knitting. If you are not willing to turn off your screens (phone, tablet, television, or computer) during your wind-down routine, consider blocking the blue light on your screen (see below). As with everything we discuss in this book, there are a lot of individual differences; we encourage you to think carefully about what activities are most likely to help you wind down and set you up for sleep. Doing crossword or Sudoku puzzles or reading an engaging novel may be just the thing to clear your mind, or it may activate you too much. Journaling may be a nice way to review your day and put it behind you, or it may stir you up.

Dim ambient lighting in the hour before bedtime.

Before electricity, humans spent most of their evenings in relative darkness. Now we spend hours after sundown in spaces illuminated by artificial light, which throws off our internal body clock. Lights send the wrong message to the brain, telling it to stay awake and stay active. For example, darkness cues your body to produce melatonin, a hormone that creates a sense of sleepiness and contributes to the architecture of your sleep cycle. Dimming or darkening your environment before bedtime will facilitate this process.

Turn off electronic devices an hour before bedtime.

Electronic devices are sleep's nemesis! They produce bright light and stimulating images, both of which are counterproductive to what your body needs to fall asleep and to stay asleep. The most optimal choice is to use these devices only during your daytime hours. If you are not ready to take a (temporary) break from electronic devices before bedtime, take precautions to block the blue light rays from your device, since blue light suppresses melatonin more than other light wavelengths. You can download apps that remove these specific light wavelengths, purchase an orange gel to put over your device, or wear blue-blocking sunglasses.

Sleep on a comfortable bed.

Comfort is a lens that will change as your body's needs change over your lifespan. Assess your bed in terms of the softness or firmness you prefer in a mattress as well as whether the mattress and your bedding provide your preferred level of warmth or coolness. Pay attention to your comfort when you sleep on other beds (such as at a hotel or at a friend's or family member's home) to identify helpful changes regarding your bed or bedding. If it isn't practical to purchase a new mattress, you may be able to add a less expensive "topper" to achieve your desired sleep surface. We do not mean to suggest that you need a "perfect" mattress; remember that we want to encourage flexibility and an ability to sleep in varying circumstances. However, we have worked with some people who were trying to sleep in a chair or on a couch, and this level of discomfort was clearly disruptive to their sleep.

Create a comfortable bedroom environment.

For most people an optimal bedroom will be dark, quiet, and well ventilated, and have a comfortable temperature. However, if you lived for years in a city, complete quiet may be so unfamiliar that you may sleep better with white noise. Notice, though, that we encourage you to use "white noise," which is consistent. If you sleep with the television or radio on, the volume will change many times a night as the broadcast moves between programs or between programming and commercials; these volume changes can pull you out of deeper stages of sleep even if they don't fully awaken you, leading to less restorative sleep.

If your environment is too noisy or light, you may want to consider using earplugs, a noise machine, or an eye mask. These inexpensive tools can be very helpful, but they can also backfire—we have worked with people who had so much ritual around creating an ideal sleep environment that this increased their stress and arousal, especially when something went awry, such as if they forgot their eye mask when traveling. Try to find the sweet spot: aim for desirable, even if not ideal, conditions, while trying to have a flexible, accepting attitude so that you will be able to adapt as conditions change.

Limit disruptions from your bed partners.

Finding a balance between your sleep needs and those of your significant other, your children, or animals is an important piece of sleep hygiene. If your partners snore, kick, are restless, hop in and out of bed, or (in the case of animals) sleep on your head, consider a trial period of sleeping alone to see if your sleep improves. You can then make an informed decision about whether the benefits of sleeping with your partner (or partners) outweigh the costs.

We commonly learn that our clients' sleep is being disturbed by their partners' snoring. If this is true for you, you may want to wear earplugs. Or, an often overlooked option is for your partner to remedy the snoring directly if this hasn't already been attempted. For example, he or she may benefit from a sleep study to assess for sleep apnea, a decongestant to treat a stuffy nose, or a modified diet to address foods sensitivities. Or perhaps you have observed that your partner only snores when sleeping on his back; he can use a positional device to help him stay on his side. Finally, if nudging your snoring partner has the desired effect, but you are hesitant to do this too often so as not to disturb his sleep, please talk to your partner; you will likely get his reassurance that it is okay to nudge as many times as you need to.

Although we have been focused on how to keep bed partners from disturbing your sleep, you also can consider asking your human bed partners to help you; getting their support to stick to your treatment program can make all the difference.

How to Make Hard Changes

Knowing what you "should" do and doing it are two very different things. Here are some of the things we want you to keep in mind as you work to improve your sleep hygiene.

Be Flexible

We strongly encourage you to think of sleep hygiene as a set of guidelines and not rigid rules. The impact that any particular behavior has on your sleep is unique to you. The guidelines are based on what we know to be true generally, or on average; they also are based entirely on what we understand about the physiology of sleep, without considering the impact of your thoughts and feelings. For example, although it is generally recommended that you not exercise strenuously in the hour before bed, one of our clients found that this was one of the best ways to prepare for bed. He told us, "I know that I am taking care of myself. This calms my brain which then calms my body." For him, the calming effect outweighed any negative impact the exercise might have had on the rhythm of his core body temperature. Similarly, it may be worth having your sleep disrupted by your cat because of the greater ease with which you fall asleep when she keeps you company in bed.

We are not encouraging you to defy the sleep hygiene guidelines just because it is easier or preferable to not change. Rather, consider each guideline and how following it more closely may impact your physiology, thoughts, and feelings, given your personal set of circumstances. Then, if you are willing, do an experiment. The client we referenced above already had sleep log data with his normal late-night exercise; he then moved his exercise to earlier in the day and continued to track his sleep. After a couple of weeks he could confidently say that moving his exercise earlier in order to be more consistent with sleep hygiene guidelines did not help his sleep—and may even have hurt it. Similarly, even if you think the benefit you derive from sleeping with your cat outweighs the cost, your cat may be disturbing your sleep more than you think, and we encourage you to collect data by doing a trial without the cat in your room.

In addition to encouraging flexibility to allow for individual differences, we also are encouraging you to remain somewhat flexible because we know that being very rigid about following a list of prescribed rules can backfire. Your life starts to revolve (even more) around your sleep and you put even more pressure on yourself to do everything "right" and to sleep *tonight*! This is counter to the work we did in chapter 4 to increase your willingness to not sleep. Remember, we want to help you hit the "sweet spot," being strict enough with yourself that you are actually doing the treatment and it has the time it needs to work, but not so strict that your anxiety increases or you cannot adapt to new situations, such as sleeping in less ideal conditions while traveling. Seeing sleep hygiene for what it is—a set of guidelines rather than rules—will help you to not respond with alarm if you "break a rule." Set some specific goals for yourself, but also remember to be flexible, based on your situation. It is likely that your priorities will shift based on whether you are at home or on vacation, under a deadline, or managing a stressful life event.

Increase Willingness

One of the biggest obstacles to changing behavior is not wanting to. The good news is that you do not have to want to do something in order to do it. For example, you may be willing to give up caffeine even though you love the boost it gives you; you may be willing to dim your lights as you approach bedtime even though you prefer a bright space. Why would you be willing to do things that you do not want to do? Usually it is because you expect to gain something. Hopefully our explanation of how sleep works and of the 3P model of insomnia (chapters 2 and 3) helped you understand that changing your behavior can break the spiral of insomnia: even though poor sleep hygiene is not likely to have caused your sleep problem, it may be maintaining it over time.

In order to increase your willingness to follow the sleep hygiene guidelines, you may want to revisit the questions we posed in chapter 4 for each behavior you are thinking of changing:

If I make this change, what will I have to give up?

If I make this change, what might I have to experience?

Am I willing to give up X?

Am I willing to have Y?

What do I hope to gain by giving up X or experiencing Y?

How important are these gains I hope to achieve?

Would it be worth it to give up X or have Y if I knew I would make these gains?

It is important to have this conversation with yourself before you are faced with making a change. That way, when your mind is feeling the urge to do what you have always done, you are prepared to do something different. Be prepared to face and refute convincing language such as *I can't give up my caffeine until I am sleeping again. It is the only thing that helps me get through my day.* This circular thinking is a common barrier, and you will be more likely to succeed if you are prepared for these types of thoughts. A helpful response could be: *Maybe this is true, but I would like to find out. I am going to give up the caffeine for three weeks to see what happens to my sleep.*

Have Realistic Expectations

Be patient. The brain is designed to make changes over time, not in a knee-jerk fashion; it may need two to four weeks of consistent data and practice (such as waking at the same time) to make a shift. In addition, you may need to follow most of the sleep hygiene guidelines before your sleep improves. If you create a wind-down routine and establish a consistent wake time, that is a great start, but it is unrealistic to expect great progress if you continue to consume energy drinks late in the day and try to sleep in an uncomfortable armchair. A comprehensive sleep hygiene program will likely be more effective than a single-component program.

Another aspect of managing expectations is to not expect sleep hygiene alone to cure your insomnia. Most people in the field of behavioral sleep medicine agree that although good sleep hygiene is important in maintaining healthy sleep, it is unlikely on its own to fix a long-standing sleep problem. This is why we encourage sleep hygiene as a way to support either stimulus control therapy or sleep restriction therapy, rather than as a stand-alone treatment. However, if your habits are very inconsistent with the sleep hygiene guidelines, it would certainly be reasonable to try sleep hygiene on its own if this is the program that you are most willing to do. We have had a few clients who needed only this treatment; they have tended to be people with very poor sleep hygiene and recent, rather than long-standing, sleep problems.

Base Decisions on Data

Keep track of what you are doing. This is an experiment, so treat it like any scientist would by keeping an objective daily record. The sleep log is an ideal tool for this. If you are working on decreasing alcohol use or having a more consistent sleep schedule, or want to see what happens if you change the time you take a medication or exercise, the sleep log will give you all the information you need to track your progress and look for any relationship between these behaviors and your sleep patterns. For other guidelines, you may need to expand on the basic sleep log directions. For example, if you implement a wind-down routine, you can create symbols to track when you engaged in your wind-down and what you did; if you experiment with having a snack before bed, you can mark when you last ate. We generally find that it is best to do this in either the "Medications" or "C-A-N-E" row, leaving the "Sleep Cycle" row uncluttered so that it is easier to see your time in bed and time asleep.

Make a Plan

For each change you are considering, make a specific plan. Your plan should include a clear definition of your goal (for example, no caffeine at all; or no caffeine after noon; or no caffeinated beverages after noon, but small amounts such as in chocolate are okay); any obstacles you anticipate (for example, craving, or lack of decaffeinated options); a plan for how to overcome those obstacles (for example, remind self of reasons for making this change; purchase decaffeinated coffee and herbal teas); and how you will track how closely you followed the guideline and the impact on your sleep (for example, using a sleep log).

Your Sleep Hygiene Plan

Worksheet 9.1 will help you develop your personal sleep hygiene plan and use the implementation tips we reviewed. You will need to refer back to the sleep hygiene questions you answered in chapter 5. You may notice that we had you write the number of days in a week that you follow the guideline, rather than just whether you do or do not follow the guideline. This is because behavior is on a continuum. If you drink alcohol before bed every night, this is different than drinking before bed once a week, for example.

This more fine-tuned measure also allows you to see incremental progress. If you drink before bed on two nights instead of your previous seven, you can see that you followed the guideline on five nights, rather than only seeing that you did not follow the guideline exactly. We hope this helps you maintain your motivation to change, and helps you strive for even greater adherence to the guidelines.

You may be wondering how many nights is "good enough." For example, if you have a consistent wake time five out of seven mornings, is that good enough? In general, we encourage you to strive to hit your target every day, especially in the beginning. Once you have established a new pattern or habit, you can experiment and collect data to see if small variations have a negative effect on your sleep. Remember to use effectiveness (what works), rather than rigid rules, to guide you.

WORKSHEET 9.1: **Your Sleep Hygiene Plan**

Use your responses to the questions in chapter 5 and the explanation of the sleep hygiene guidelines in this chapter to complete this worksheet.

STEP 1: Rate how IMPORTANT you think it is, how WILLING you are, and how CONFIDENT you are that you will be able to continue to follow the guidelines you already are following. Then do the same for the guidelines you are not closely following. Use a scale of 0–10:

0		5		10
Not at all	A little	Somewhat	Quite	Extremely or completely

Sleep Hygiene Guidelines I Am Already Following Closely:

	How I Feel About Continuing to Follow This Guideline		
Guideline	**Importance of**	**Willingness to**	**Confidence I Can**
Sample *Consistent wake time*	8	10	10

Sleep Hygiene Guidelines I am NOT Following Closely:

	How I Feel About Continuing to Follow This Guideline		
Guideline	Importance of	Willingness to	Confidence I Can
Sample Consistent bedtime	9	6	4

STEP 2: Next, make a plan for each guideline you rated as IMPORTANT but (a) are not now following, or (b) have low confidence you will continue to follow. If you need more room, you can download additional copies of this worksheet from http://www.newharbinger.com/33438. Here is a sample.

Guideline	*Wind-Down Routine*
My Goal	*Listen to music on back porch with lights turned down. Start with fifteen minutes; increase to thirty minutes after three to four days.*
Why Important	*Will quiet my mind, relax me, and help my body clock transition from wake to sleep.*
Willingness	What will I have to give up? *Time to get something done; spontaneity* What will I have to experience? *Guilt (So much to do. How can I just relax?)* Why am I willing despite this? *Insomnia is costing me a lot, including being unproductive and inefficient at times. If I give up fifteen to thirty minutes for a wind-down period, I may get more, not less, done. I don't actually believe I'm bad for relaxing for fifteen to thirty minutes, so I don't have to listen to my guilt. I'll do this as an experiment. If it costs me too much, I can always go back to my old habit.*
Obstacles and Solutions	*O: Will lose track of time and suddenly it will be bedtime. S: Set alarm for forty minutes before target bedtime.* *O: My mind will tell me to do "just this one thing." S: Remind myself why I am willing; remind myself that I already know how things have been going without a wind-down, and want to try something different; I'll do that "one thing" tomorrow.*
How to Track	*Write in C-A-N-E row of sleep log.*

Guideline	
My Goal	
Why Important	
Willingness	What will I have to give up? What will I have to experience? Why am I willing despite this?
Obstacles and Solutions	
How to Track	

Guideline	
My Goal	
Why Important	
Willingness	What will I have to give up? What will I have to experience? Why am I willing despite this?
Obstacles and Solutions	
How to Track	

Guideline	
My Goal	
Why Important	
Willingness	What will I have to give up? What will I have to experience? Why am I willing despite this?
Obstacles and Solutions	
How to Track	

Guideline	
My Goal	
Why Important	
Willingness	What will I have to give up? What will I have to experience? Why am I willing despite this?
Obstacles and Solutions	
How to Track	

Summary of Part 2

BEHAVIORAL STRATEGIES

At this point in the program, you have created your personal behavioral sleep program. You have determined if you are willing and ready to engage in stimulus control therapy, sleep restriction therapy, or a combined program. You also have assessed your unique sleep hygiene needs and determined if you are willing to make some behavioral or environmental changes to support restorative sleep. You may even be some weeks into your behavioral program. You may be returning again and again to willingness skills to optimize your behavioral programs. Hopefully you are continuing to keep a sleep log so you can track your progress.

Behavioral programs are the heart of cognitive behavioral therapy for insomnia and are key to your success. Still, research tells us that adding cognitive therapy may increase your success (Harvey et al., 2014). Cognitive strategies can help you to harness the power your mind has over your body and your behavioral choices. The next section is dedicated to these strategies. Go ahead and turn the page. We will see you there!

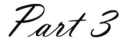

Part 3

Cognitive Strategies

This next section is dedicated to your thoughts and how they impact your sleep. You may recall from chapter 3 that there are numerous factors that can tip the scale from restorative sleep to nonrestorative sleep. In these next three chapters, we focus on how your thoughts weigh in on this scale.

The first two chapters in this section, chapters 10 and 11, will teach you two cognitive strategies used in traditional CBT-I. These strategies are change-based interventions. Change-based strategies teach you how to change the content and the timing of your thoughts. In chapter 10 we focus on *what* you are thinking. We review how negative thought patterns interfere with your sleep. We also provide a tool for managing these negative cognitions. In chapter 11 we will help you change *when* you are thinking, so a busy mind does not keep you up at night.

In chapter 12, we teach you two additional cognitive skills: mindfulness and cognitive defusion. These are acceptance-based interventions that depart from the change model in chapters 10 and 11. Acceptance-based interventions focus on the way your mind responds to your thoughts, as opposed to altering the thoughts themselves. These skills are not a part of traditional CBT-I. We borrow them from acceptance and commitment therapy in order to optimize CBT-I.

You are welcome to read these chapters in sequence and make use of all of the strategies. If you prefer to focus your efforts on just one or two strategies, look back at the work you did in chapter 5 and on worksheet 5.1. Which strategies seemed most relevant? With which did you say you would start? Go ahead and skip to that chapter now.

Chapter 10

Changing What You Think (Cognitive Restructuring)

*I*t is estimated that humans produce hundreds, if not thousands, of thoughts per hour. This staggering amount of information is designed to help you make sense of the world. Thoughts come from countless sources, including your observations, your expectations, and your own personal experiences. Your mind uses categories and labels to sort through and organize all of this information. Your mind groups your thoughts and uses themes like good/bad, always/never, right/wrong, and love/hate. Check in with your mind now. What are your thoughts? Perhaps you are noticing your curiosity about this chapter. Maybe you are thinking about how you slept last night. See if you can identify how your mind categorized these thoughts. Perhaps you labeled your curiosity as "helpful" and your sleep last night as "problematic." Take a moment or two to consider the content of your thoughts.

Minds are not 100% accurate. Nor do they only produce helpful thoughts. Minds are often even less accurate and less helpful when they are sleepy or feeling strong emotions. For example, if you are exhausted and concerned about your sleep, you may be more likely to have thoughts like *I am never going to sleep tonight!* Of course, this thought just feeds the insomnia spiral. You experience an unpleasant emotional reaction such as frustration or hopelessness. These feelings then activate your nervous system, telling it that something is wrong. This sends a signal to your body to be more alert so that it can attend to the problematic situation. This, of course, makes it harder to sleep.

Who Should Use Cognitive Restructuring?

Cognitive restructuring (CR) can help you change myths about what "normal" sleep is, catastrophic thoughts about what will happen if you do not sleep, negative thoughts about other things in your life that increase stress or anxiety, and thoughts that interfere with your willingness to change sleep-related behaviors. Here are some clues that cognitive restructuring will likely be useful for you:

- You have a lot of "should" or "must" notions about sleep (such as: *I should be able to fall asleep within five minutes*; *I must sleep tonight*; or *I should sleep through the night without interruption*).

- You are very concerned about how your insomnia is affecting your health or functioning.

- You have intrusive or anxiety-provoking thoughts about your sleep.

- You think that stress, anxiety, or depression is adding to your sleep problems.

- You believe that you are not capable of making a behavioral change you think would be helpful.

- You believe that behavioral strategies will not help your insomnia.

Negative Cognitions

Negative cognitions are thoughts that are either distorted or unhelpful (or both). Negative cognitions activate your body and interfere with your wake and sleep cycles. Negative cognitions also increase discomfort. They make it more likely that you will choose short-term solutions for your sleep. They make it less likely that you will make choices that support sustainable sleep patterns in the long term. They have a disruptive impact on your sleep. They feed your insomnia spiral.

There are three things you need to know about negative thoughts. First, it is normal to have negative thoughts about your sleep. Negative thoughts are a very human response to a challenging situation. Second, negative thoughts tend to increase when you are sleepy or are feeling strong emotions. Most people who struggle with sleep have lots of negative thoughts about sleep. Third, negative thoughts feed negative thoughts. Once a thought shows up, it will cue another negative thought, and another. Therefore, negative thoughts are expected, but they also contribute to your insomnia. This is why cognitive strategies are such an important part of CBT-I.

Cognitive Distortions

One type of negative thought is a distorted thought. Distortion literally means an alteration of the original state. A cognitive distortion, then, is a thought that has a kernel of truth in it, but has been altered in some way. Cognitive distortions misrepresent the situations they describe. For example, you may say "I didn't sleep a wink last night," when you actually slept for a few hours.

There are recurring themes in the manner in which our minds distort our thoughts. Below is a list of common types of cognitive distortions. Read the descriptions and see which you engage in most often.

All-or-nothing thinking. This is when your mind forces a choice between all or nothing. Perhaps you eat a cookie after you told yourself no. You have the thought, *There goes my diet. I might as well eat them all.* Your mind is engaging in all-or-nothing thinking.

Catastrophizing. This is when you think that you will not be able to cope with something bad happening. You are worried you will not perform well giving a presentation and you think, *I will just die of embarrassment.* Your mind is engaging in catastrophizing.

Overgeneralization. This is when your mind views one event as representative of all events. If you fall down once while skiing and think, *I'll never be able to ski this run,* your mind is engaging in overgeneralization.

Mental filtering. This is when your mind dwells on the negatives and ignores the positives. You get a 99% on a test. You have the thought, *What did I do wrong?* Your mind is using a distorted mental filter in noticing the one point missed instead of the ninety-nine earned.

Labeling. This is when your mind attaches a label or story to a person or situation. You make an embarrassing comment in front of someone. Your mind tells you, *You are such a loser!* Your mind is engaging in unhelpful labeling.

Personalization and blaming. This happens when your mind assigns fault. You feel bad that a friend did not like your book recommendation. You have the thought, *It's my fault; I* *should have known better*. Your mind is using personalization. Another example: you feel angry that a friend did not recommend a good book to you. You have the thought, *That person is a bad friend; he should know me better than that*. Your mind is engaging in the use of inaccurate blame.

Cognitive distortions can be about any topic and still impact your sleep. In fact, none of the examples of cognitive distortions listed above are about sleep. Yet they share a common tone of judgment and blame. This can increase your arousal and negatively impact your ability to fall asleep and stay asleep.

Unhelpful Cognitions

A second type of negative thought is an unhelpful cognition. Unhelpful cognitions are thoughts that, regardless of how accurate or distorted they are, have a negative impact on you. An example of a nondistorted but unhelpful cognition about sleep is *Even if I fall asleep right now, I will only get five hours of sleep!* This thought may be true, but it is also counterproductive because it produces emotional responses (such as anxiety and frustration) that interfere with what your body needs for sleep.

Cognitive Restructuring

There is an effective tool for managing these negative cognitions. It is known as "cognitive restructuring," which literally means changing or restoring the content of your thoughts. Cognitive restructuring helps you strip away distortions, leaving you with more accurate thoughts. Cognitive restructuring also helps you recognize accurate but unhelpful thoughts. There are three steps to cognitive restructuring, and we will look at each in turn:

- Identify the thought(s).

- Challenge the thought(s).

- Use your alternative thought(s) to generate alternative action.

1. Identify the thoughts.

You may be quite aware of the thoughts that are causing you distress and feeding the insomnia cycle. If you are, go ahead and write them down. Then move on to step 2.

However, many people are not exactly sure what is going through their minds. Oftentimes, thoughts are so quick and automatic we are unaware of them.

"Thought records" are a tool designed to help you become more skilled at identifying and working with your thoughts. Worksheet 10.1 is a version that we like. We encourage you to use a spike in emotions to help you identify your negative thoughts. When you notice such a spike, first list the feelings you just noticed (for example, "fear" or "dread") in the third column. Then write in the first column a very brief explanation of the situation (for example, "Preparing for bed"). Then ask yourself, *What was going through my mind?* and write your thoughts in the second column (for example, "What if I don't sleep tonight?").

Here are a couple of hints to help you with step 1. First, try to capture your thoughts precisely as you said them to yourself. The way you talk to yourself really does matter. A thought like *I'm such an idiot!* will affect you very differently than the thought *I sure made a mistake!* Second, consider whether the thoughts you identified are specific enough to work with. If they are lacking in detail, it can be helpful to dig deeper. Start with the thought that showed up, and then ask yourself, *And then what?* in order to get more information. For example, the thought *I am scared I won't be good at my presentation tomorrow if I don't sleep tonight* is activating but lacking detail. Are you worrying about failure? Job security? Judgment from colleagues? Once you have more details, you have a greater capacity to work with your cognitive distortions or unhelpful thoughts.

2. Challenge the thoughts.

The next step in this process is to spot the "negative" in your thought. This can be tricky, and referring to the list of distortions can help you. With the thought *I'll never get to sleep*, the distortion is the word "never," because it is not physically possible to never sleep. Sleep is required to live, and eventually your sleep drive will win out and force your body to rest. The data to support the thought is not there; no one on this planet has lived without sleeping. The data against the thought is strong: eventually you will fall asleep. You now modify the original thought to strip away the distortion, while leaving the kernel of truth: *I struggle to get to sleep*, or *Getting to sleep is really hard for me*, or *I am afraid that I won't ever sleep*. These thoughts, without the distortion, are painful but not absolute. They will naturally have a different influence on your emotions and behaviors than the thought that contains the word "never."

3. Use your alternative thoughts to generate alternative action.

The final step in our thought record is to consider: What next? Take a look at your alternative thoughts and notice if your emotions and physical sensations have changed. If yes, how have they changed? What are your feelings now? What are your options now? We believe that alternative thoughts will allow you to recognize the option of alternative behaviors. If your thought has been modified from *I'll never get to sleep* to *I am afraid that I won't ever sleep*, what shows up? Perhaps your emotions have shifted from fear to sadness or frustration. Perhaps the recognition is that yes, sleep is currently challenging for you. You can recognize that you are addressing this issue by reading sleep books and trying new techniques for your sleep. Your alternative behavior could be to reach for your personalized sleep program to remind yourself of what actions you are taking to improve the quality of your sleep. The goal in this step is to lessen the amount of control your negative cognitions have on your actions. If you look back at the 3P model in figure 3.1, you will see how this can interrupt the insomnia spiral.

Example: George's Cognitive Restructuring

Remember George from chapter 3? He is a self-employed businessman whose sleep problems started after the birth of his third child. His current difficulties include trouble falling asleep and waking too early in the morning (around 3 a.m.). He is fatigued during the day, concerned about his job productivity, and anxious about how to fix his sleep problems. Take a look at worksheet 10.1 to see how George would complete a thought record. Some key thoughts are acknowledged. These thoughts are then challenged and replaced. Finally, alternative actions are identified.

WORKSHEET 10.1: Cognitive Restructuring Thought Record

Date _____

STEP 1: Awareness		STEP 2: Challenge		STEP 3: What Next?
What is the situation?	What is your thought? Be specific and identify each one separately.	What are your feelings?	Can you find any distortion? If yes, what is it and what is the more accurate thought?	Is the thought unhelpful? If yes, what is a more helpful thought?	What are your feelings now? How does challenging your thoughts influence your choices?

Sample: George

STEP 1: Awareness			STEP 2: Challenge		STEP 3: What Next?
What is the situation?	What is your thought? Be specific and identify each one separately.	What are your feelings?	Can you find any distortion? If yes, what is it and what is the more accurate thought?	Is the thought unhelpful? If yes, what is a more helpful thought?	What are your feelings now? How does challenging your thoughts influence your choices?
Tossing and turning at bedtime.	I will fail at my job tomorrow.	Panic, anger.	Distortion: I will fail. Accurate: It may be more difficult to do my job.	Very unhelpful to think I will fail. More helpful to recognize it might be harder to do my job.	Frustration and acceptance. I do not like having to work harder, but it is my reality at this time. Settle down.
Waking up multiple times during the night.	This insomnia is killing me.	Fear, sadness.	Distortion: killing me. Accurate: challenging and painful. I will not die from this insomnia.	Yes, unhelpful. More helpful to know sleep is challenging right now.	Determination. I am ready to do what it takes to change my relationship with sleep.
Fatigue and "fog" during my business presentation.	I am a failure.	Disgust, embarrassment.	Distortion: I = failure. Accurate: I am struggling with this presentation right now.	Very unhelpful to label myself and all I do as a failure. More helpful to recognize this is a tough time.	Concern and anxiety. I will need to take some extra time and care to make sure I am running my business as best I can.

Challenging Common Cognitive Distortions About Sleep

Here are some common cognitive distortions specifically about sleep. Do any of these sound familiar? Notice how we challenge these thoughts. Can you consider these alternative thoughts?

"I can't do anything to improve my sleep."

It is true that many sleep-interfering factors are partially out of your control, such as pain, allergies, menopause, and depression. But there are also many factors that are under your control. These controllable factors include lifestyles, unhelpful habits, and stress management. Removing this distortion can help you to identify what you can control. Focus on the areas of your life that are open for change. This book highlights all that you *can* do to improve your sleep.

"I should be able to sleep whenever and however I want to."

No one has this type of control and consistency. In fact, no two nights of sleep are really alike. There are natural and daily fluctuations in sleep, just as with your appetite and mood. Nobody has control over when they fall asleep and wake up. Eight hours of sleep is an average, not a given.

"I have to work harder at my sleep."

This pressure perpetuates a tug of war with the Insomnia Monster. You will find your sweet spot with sleep when you determine when to work harder and when to let go of the rope.

"I have to make sleep happen right now."

This puts you at risk for getting trapped in an ineffective spiral, just like the Chinese finger traps. This creates anxiety, as well as a "fix it" attitude, at a time when your brain would instead benefit from some willingness.

How Cognitive Restructuring Can Go Awry

Sometimes people misunderstand our intent when we introduce cognitive restructuring. They think we are suggesting that they "think positively," or that they control their mind and stop having negative thoughts. If this is how you try to work with your thoughts, chances are you will simply increase your struggle. Instead, we encourage you to use your willingness skills as you work with your thoughts. Can you be willing to have whatever thoughts show up, but then choose to respond differently to them?

Regarding the "think positively" misconception, it is common to feel pressure to generate new thoughts that are optimistic and hopeful. It makes sense that people think this is what cognitive restructuring is about, since the brain is designed to categorize, and the opposite of negative is positive. However, we actually are encouraging you to go from negative to realistic, not from unrealistically negative to unrealistically positive. If an optimistic, hopeful thought is truly a realistic appraisal, then all is well and your mind will be pleased to know this information. However, if this is an example of forcing a positive attitude, it will most likely backfire. You will not believe it. It will not work. Your mind will see right through you! It is far more effective to remove all distortion, even the positive. This often requires leaning into (rather than resisting) some discomfort. This takes some willingness to resist the urge to replace all your negative thoughts with positive ones.

The second misconception is thinking that you have to stop having certain thoughts. Because of the way our brains are wired, this is simply not possible. Yet you might find yourself with thoughts such as *Stop thinking that way!* and *You must think positively!* We want you to recognize that this is really just another form of negative thought patterns! It is both unhelpful and distorted—no one can control what thoughts enter their mind, and no one is capable of positive thoughts 100% of the time. Consider these alternative thoughts: *I am doing the best I can by noticing my thoughts and their content. The goal is not to get rid of thoughts, but rather to catch them in action and provide a more viable alternative thought.* As you practice cognitive restructuring, be sure not to fight your mind. Instead, simultaneously practice willingness for all types of thoughts to exist in your mind. And then use your alternative thought to guide effective action.

Common Questions (and Answers)

"I do not have any thoughts that interfere with my sleep. Do I really need to keep a thought record?"

It is most likely that you do have thoughts that interfere with your sleep but that you are unaware of them. Thoughts can be very tricky. It can be difficult to notice them. Use your body for clues that you may be engaging in negative thinking. If you notice tension, discomfort, or strong emotions, these will be linked to important thoughts. You can take a close look at the thoughts that you identify in this manner to see if they are distorted or unhelpful.

"I do not have my thought record sheet with me. Should I track my thoughts anyway?"

The worksheet is there to help guide you in the process of cognitive restructuring, and to serve as a reminder to work on this skill. If you do not have a copy of the worksheet with you, go ahead and use whatever is close and handy. Some other options include index cards, paper, journals, or a cocktail napkin! It is fine to create your own version of a thought record. As long as you have a way to track, you will find benefit in this intervention.

"I cannot figure out how my thought is unhelpful. What do I do now?"

It is possible that you are actually trying to challenge more than one thought at once. What happens if you break down a complex thought into parts, and treat each part as a separate thought? It will be easier to spot the unhelpful elements when you look at one idea at a time.

If you find you are still struggling with uncovering the unhelpful parts of your thought, ask yourself this question: "And then what?" This line of questioning will also help you to break down thoughts and get to their core. For example, let's say you feel anxious and your thought is: *I am so tired.* The thought is not distorted—you are tired. Yet it is not immediately clear why this thought would make you anxious. One could be relieved to be tired. Probe further. *Okay, I am tired. Now what? What is the worst that could happen?* Asking yourself these questions can help you get to the distorted thought, such as *I can't stand it!* or *I am sure to mess up when I am this tired.*

"Are you sure this intervention will help me?"

No. But we suspect it will. Using the thought record to monitor what you are thinking will help you better understand what your mind tells you about sleep. It also may help to create some distance between you and your thoughts (there is much more on this in chapter 12). Catching and correcting distorted thoughts may decrease your arousal and your struggle with sleep. This is not a guarantee that it will solve all your sleep challenges. It is simply an acknowledgment that cognitive restructuring is a powerful tool.

"Do I have to do the thought record every day?"

We encourage you to complete at least one thought record a day at first, just to get skilled at recognizing thoughts and their connection to your feelings. After that, use the thought record in response to strong emotional reactions, or when you are aware that you are thinking about your sleep or the cost of your insomnia.

"I keep trying to replace my negative thoughts with positive thoughts. Why can't I convince my brain to be more optimistic?"

The goal of restructuring is not to generate positive thoughts. The goal is to look for unhelpful patterns that are hiding in your thoughts. When you restructure these unhelpful thoughts, you want to replace them with more workable, more accurate thoughts. Sometimes these new thoughts are positive. More often they are not. However, the accuracy allows you to have a more clear understanding of your situation, which will better guide effective action.

"Now that I understand how these negative thoughts impact my sleep, I need them to stop. How can I only have helpful thoughts about sleep?"

You can't. Stopping thoughts is not the goal of cognitive restructuring. We have learned that trying to stop or suppress thoughts can lead to more distress, not less. These negative thoughts are habits. It takes time and practice to make new habits. However, even after you have developed new habits, you will still have negative thoughts. What will be different will be your habits about how you manage or respond to these negative thoughts.

"I am feeling overwhelmed and lost in this process."

If the thought record feels overwhelming, consider doing a thought record around the thought record! Seriously. Something important is showing up. Are you placing too much pressure on yourself by forcing yourself to push harder than is comfortable? Perhaps slowing down could be the most supportive move. Are you uncovering some really important and big feelings about sleep and your life? Perhaps talking to someone such as a friend or trained clinician can benefit you at this time. Remember, the intensity of your reaction is providing you with important information.

Are you trying to monitor too many of your thoughts? We are not suggesting that you write everything down! Focus on the thoughts that seem to be connected to your sleep. These are most likely predictions about how you will sleep, thoughts about what it will mean if you do not sleep well, or thoughts about stressful life events that have your body "wired." Or focus on thoughts that are blocking you from fully implementing a behavioral sleep program.

Your Cognitive Restructuring Plan

Use worksheet 10.1 to start working with your distorted or unhelpful thoughts. Spend some time considering what types of thoughts tend to feed your insomnia spiral. Identify your thoughts about sleep. Identify your thoughts about your life more generally that also impact your sleep patterns. Remember to look out for the four most common targets of cognitive restructuring: (1) myths about what normal sleep is like, (2) catastrophic thoughts about what will happen if you do not sleep, (3) negative thoughts about other things in your life that increase stress or anxiety, and (4) thoughts that interfere with your willingness to change sleep-related behaviors. Keep in mind that bodily sensations and strong emotions can help you to uncover important thoughts.

Pay attention to your thoughts every day. It will take time and practice to help your brain catch and change the problematic patterns. Use your willingness skills to lean into your experience, even as you challenge your thoughts. Be careful not to have cognitive restructuring add to your struggle.

What to Expect

You can expect to still have negative thoughts. You are human. Humans have inaccurate thoughts every day. The goal is not to get rid of certain types of thoughts. The goal is to decrease the impact of these negative thoughts on your sleep and well-being.

You can expect to see a change in how you respond to your negative thoughts. You will become more aware of the thoughts. You will be more likely to pause. You will be less likely to take your thoughts at face value. You will notice yourself fact-checking, asking questions such as *Are there any distortions lurking in this thought?*

With practice you will get quicker and quicker at identifying and replacing negative cognitions. You likely will see patterns in the type of negative thoughts your mind generates. This will allow you to challenge similar thoughts much more quickly. For example, you may say to yourself, *Oh, there I go catastrophizing again. I know I will survive.*

Over time, you may notice that you have fewer negative cognitions to challenge. Or you may not. Either way, this process of pausing, questioning, and restructuring will help you step out of the insomnia spiral. You will find yourself using your more accurate and helpful thoughts to inform your behavioral decisions. As a result, your ability to stick to your behavioral program will improve. You also will notice less physiological arousal as you change your self-talk.

How to Evaluate Your Progress and When to Consider a Different Strategy

There are no clear, quantifiable measures of progress with cognitive restructuring. Use effectiveness as your compass. Is it getting easier to notice and challenge negative thoughts? Does changing the way you are thinking help to calm your mind and nervous system so that you feel less anxiety, tension, or other distress? Does challenging negative thoughts help you stick to your behavioral program?

If you have completed many thought records over the course of several weeks and perceive no benefit at all, we encourage you to try the other cognitive strategies in this book. You may also want to take a break from cognitive restructuring if this tool is having the undesirable effect of getting you really "caught up" in your head. Ideally, cognitive restructuring will give you some distance from your negative thoughts and allow you to gain a more realistic perspective. Occasionally people have the opposite experience. This is not effective.

Your Next Step

If you are finding cognitive restructuring helpful, continue to use this tool in addition to working your behavioral sleep program. You can pause here, and put your time and effort into these treatment components. Then, once you have been following your behavioral program for at least six to eight weeks, you are welcome to skip to chapter 13 to evaluate your progress thus far.

Alternatively, you can add to your arsenal of cognitive strategies. Refer back to worksheet 5.1 to remind yourself which other cognitive strategies seemed relevant to you. Then proceed to either chapter 11 to learn about designated worry time, or chapter 12 to learn about the acceptance-based strategies of mindfulness and cognitive defusion.

Chapter 11

Changing When and Where You Think (Designated Worry Time)

*I*n the previous chapter, we focused on helping you change *what* you think. For example, you might change a really alarming thought (such as *I won't survive tomorrow if I don't get a good night's sleep tonight!*) to a less alarming and more accurate thought (such as *I'll be uncomfortable and I may not perform at my best, but I will survive tomorrow no matter how I sleep tonight*). But what if your thoughts are realistic, but you have a *lot* of them while lying in bed, such as thinking of all the items you want to get at the grocery store tomorrow, mentally preparing for a meeting, thinking fondly of memories from your youth, or working on a problem that has thus far defied solution? Or what if you have realistic thoughts again, and again, and again, when you are wanting to sleep (*I'm going to be okay. I'm going to be okay. I'm going to be okay…*)? An active mind can interfere with sleep regardless of what you are thinking. In this chapter and the next, we will focus more on your thought *process*, or *how* you are thinking, particularly when you would rather be sleeping.

Who Should Use Designated Worry Time?

This strategy will be most useful if:

- You worry a lot throughout the day; or

- Your mind is busy when you want to be sleeping. It may be busy with worry, or with other types of thoughts, such as problem-solving or planning.

Designated Worry Time for Chronic Worriers

Designated worry time (DWT) was initially developed for people with chronic worry (a condition called generalized anxiety disorder). If you are a worrier, you may think that you cannot possibly benefit from *more* worry time! However, DWT allows you to worry in a very different way. In DWT you focus only on your worries; you do not try to "talk yourself down" by giving yourself reassurance, nor do you seek reassurance from others, distract yourself, or use other techniques designed to decrease your worry. Instead, you fully immerse yourself in your worries. Another part of this immersion is that you "worry to death" one worry before moving on to the next, rather than jumping from worry to worry as chronic worriers often do. This complete immersion into your worries generally leads to a decrease in the amount of anxiety you feel when thinking about your worries (a process called *habituation*). After practicing DWT for several days, you may even be bored instead of anxious! Finally, with DWT you learn to more effectively delay worry at other times of the day or night, keeping worry more contained and less pervasive. DWT has been shown to significantly decrease worry symptoms and insomnia symptoms (McGowan & Behar, 2013).

Designated Worry Time for Insomnia

You may benefit from DWT even if you are not a chronic worrier. For example, perhaps you do not worry throughout the day, but only at night. Often we are so "on the go"—or so good at distracting ourselves—during the day that our minds do not have a lot of time to go wherever they want to go. When you get in bed and there is relative quiet, your mind may take advantage of this opportunity and worry, worry, worry. Or perhaps it is not worry but other types of thought processes that keep you awake: for example, you may lie in bed planning, reminiscing about the past, or turning a problem over in your mind seeking a creative solution. You can use the DWT paradigm to move any type of thought process to another time of day. For simplicity's sake we will mostly use the word "worry" in this chapter, but feel free to replace this with "planning" or "reminiscing" or "problem-solving" or any other term that better describes what your mind does at night.

How to Use Designated Worry Time

Regardless of whether you worry throughout the day or only at night, there are two essential components of DWT. First, you set aside time to worry earlier in the day or evening. Then, when you are worrying (or planning or reminiscing or problem-solving) at other times, you remind yourself: *Mind, you can absolutely worry about this, but this isn't the time. I gave you an opportunity to worry earlier today, and I promise to give you another opportunity tomorrow.*

Let us look at these two components in detail.

Step 1: Schedule Worry Time

- Pick one or two times a day and dedicate ten to thirty minutes to worrying. (Ten minutes is a good starting prescription. You can increase the time if you repeatedly find that this is not enough.)

- Set a timer.

- During your DWT, *only* worry. Do not problem-solve, plan, or try to reassure yourself. Do not try to distract yourself with other thoughts or activities.

- Ask yourself what you are worried about. When one worry comes to mind, really worry about that one worry. Stick with it. Ask yourself: *What about this worries me most? What's the worst that can happen?* Remember, do not problem-solve or reassure yourself that the worst possible outcome is unlikely to occur. Before moving on to the next worry, ask yourself if there are any other concerns related to *this* worry. (That is, "worry it to death.") If not, you can move on to another worry. Repeat this step until the end of your worry period.

- If you run out of worries before the timer goes off, repeat the worries you already worried to death. It is important to keep at it for the entire worry period.

- At the end of your designated worry time, you may want to take a few deep breaths, paying attention to each breath. This will help you get out of your mind and drop into your body. Then shift your focus to an activity in the present moment (for example, make dinner, engage in conversation, or do some work). The mindfulness strategies discussed in the next chapter may help with this.

Step 2: Delay Worry

- At all other times of day, *notice* when you are worrying. (*Oh, there is worry.*)

- Then, *validate.* (*I can absolutely worry about this.*)

- *Delay* to your next scheduled worry period. (*And, I have set aside time to do so. I will worry about this at 5:15 this evening.* Or: *And, I have already done so today. I will have another chance tomorrow.*)

- *Refocus* your attention on something else.

- Repeat the above steps as often as needed, even if just minutes apart!

Common Questions (and Answers)

"But I worry about real problems! I can't just stick my head in the sand and keep delaying!"

You can absolutely think about the topics of your worry at other times of the day, as long as you are actively working on the issue—by planning, researching, consulting, problem-solving, or taking action—rather than worrying. We can define "worry" as tormenting or harassing yourself with concerns about the future. When you notice that you are worrying, you really have three options: (1) continue to focus on this particular concern, but shift from worrying to taking action to address the concern; (2) delay worry to your designated time; or (3) go ahead and do your DWT.

"I seem to feel a lot worse after my worry period."

Each and every time a client has reported this, we have discovered that he or she was ruminating rather than worrying during the worry period. Although we said that you can use the DWT paradigm to help with any type of thought process that is interfering with sleep, rumination requires special attention.

Ruminating, in cognitive behavioral terms, is when you review the past again and again. While rumination is about the past, worry is about the future. For some reason, when you immerse yourself in worry, this leads to satiation or habituation, whereas immersing yourself in rumination breeds more rumination.

Do *not* use this strategy to ruminate about the past! It is fine to think about a past event, but then focus on the future consequences; do not replay the past event again and again. For example, during DWT you can think about a gaffe you made at a staff meeting the day before, but then focus on your fears about that gaffe (*My coworkers will not respect me anymore, my supervisor will not trust me with larger projects, I will be relegated to the rank and file and will never move up in the company and eventually I will be laid off and I will not be able to get another job and…*). To help you understand this difference even further, here is an example of what ruminating might sound like in the same scenario: *I can't believe I said that! How stupid of me. What did John say right before that?* [Replays the entire dialogue of the five minutes before and after the "stupid" comment.] *The look on Carrie's face…she was so surprised by what I said; she looked so disapproving. Of course, this is one of many stupid things I have said in my professional life. Like that staff meeting a couple of months ago when…*

In short, if, after several days of DWT you feel worse, there is a good chance you are ruminating. See if you can think about exactly the same issues, but focus on your fears for the future. If you think ruminating is the specific type of thought process that gets in the way of your sleep, you can still try DWT but instead of saying to yourself, *You can ruminate about this later,* when you are trying to delay, you might want to say something like: *You can think about this later; ruminating just doesn't help.*

"Can I use DWT only on days that I am more worried or anxious, instead of every day?"

DWT is most effective when practiced daily over a period of time (weeks, not just days). You may at some point graduate to using DWT only "as needed," but when you start, try to do it daily, even if you are not particularly worried on a given day. Remember that you may not be aware of worries that are percolating in the back of your mind until you slow down; better to slow down at your designated worry time than to wait until bedtime. Also, if you do not have a lot to worry about even once you slow down, this is good information for your mind to register. Then, if worries come to mind when you are in bed, you can remind yourself that by the light of day you did not even have enough worries to fill ten minutes! Plus, it is easier to delay worry if you really keep your commitment to yourself and set aside time to worry every single day. Your mind will quickly rebel if you keep telling it you will "worry tomorrow" but then rarely do.

"When I lie in bed awake I tend to think about all the things on my 'To Do' list. I do not really worry about them, I just remember or brainstorm: 'Oh, I have to schedule that doctor's appointment. Hmm, what do I need to do to get ready for my trip next week?' How do I apply DWT to this?"

During your designated time you will ask your mind to generate or review your "To Do" list. If this does not fill the entire ten minutes, you can review your list again and again until the timer goes off. You may decide to write out your list. This may help you delay when you start to cycle through your list while you are in bed. (*Thanks, mind, for reminding me of all of these important things I have to do, but I have already thought of them and put them on a list. Now is not the time to be thinking about these things. I will have another chance tomorrow.*)

"I am afraid: what if I start to worry and cannot stop?"

While this is a common concern, especially for our highly anxious clients, in our experience DWT does not "open a floodgate" that then cannot be closed. Remember that during DWT you are worrying about things that are already on your mind. You are not creating "monsters in the closet," but merely turning on the lights and looking them right in their eyes. Still, if this is a concern, we do suggest that you take steps to make it easier to shift away from your worries at the end of your worry time. First, set an alarm to help pull you out of your reverie. Second, have a specific plan for what you will do right after your worry time (for example, walk the dog, or make a phone call). Third, be prepared to start the second step of DWT immediately; if you are still worrying, remind yourself that you just had your worry time and will have another soon.

"Can I do my worry time right before bed?"

We generally recommend against this and instead suggest a buffer between your worry time and your bedtime. In fact, some people find that doing it any time in the evening is detrimental to their sleep, and find it best to do DWT earlier in the day. Others benefit from doing it in the evening, but at least two hours before bedtime. However, occasionally people find that it does help to do it just before bed; these people usually experience DWT as a "worry dump" and say that they have the clearest, most worry-free mind just after their worry period. Finally, some people will get out of bed to do their worry time if worries are keeping them awake, especially if they did not do their worry time earlier that day. We suggest you start by scheduling your worry time earlier in the day or evening and see how you respond. You can always experiment with different times of day to see what is optimal for you. Remember to use effectiveness as your compass.

"Do I need to have my worry time at the same time each day?"

No. As long as you do it, it does not matter if you do your planned worrying at the same time each day. However, you may find that it is easier to remember or easier to fit worry time into your schedule if you anchor it to a time of day (for example, 11:30 a.m.) or daily event (for example, before lunch). If this does not work for your schedule, an alternative is to enter your worry time into your calendar for the next week or so. Knowing when you will next worry will make it easier for you to delay to your next designated time.

"I do worry a lot during the day, but I do not think that worry is keeping me awake at night. I have light, fitful sleep, but I am not lying awake worrying. Can this strategy still help my sleep?"

Absolutely! If you are worrying a lot during the day, then any strategy that helps you better manage that worry can help you be less physically aroused, which can help you sleep better.

"I am skeptical."

Many of the strategies in this book are counterintuitive, and DWT is no exception. Some people think it's a brilliant concept and embrace it immediately, whereas others cannot imagine benefiting from it. One of the reasons we love this strategy is that we have an extremely high success rate with it. The only times DWT has not helped a client we were treating have been when the client did not do it, or the client ruminated during the designated time (see above). Even if you are skeptical, we encourage you to experiment by doing DWT consistently for one or two weeks. If it isn't useful, you can always stop.

Your Designated Worry Time Plan

Take some time to complete worksheet 11.1. This worksheet guides you in personalizing DWT based on your unique circumstances. If you answer yes to the last question, which asks if you are willing to try this strategy, then you are ready to start!

WORKSHEET 11.1: **Your Designated Worry Time Plan**

Designated Worry Time: Basic Recipe

1. Schedule ten to thirty minutes of worry time each day.

    *   Set a timer.

    *   Only worry. Do not problem-solve or reassure yourself.

    *   "Worry to death" one concern before moving on to another.

    *   Keep worrying for the entire worry period.

    *   At the end of your worry period, shift your focus.

    *   Use this for any thought process that interferes with sleep (for example, planning; reminiscing; problem-solving), except for rumination.

2. At all other times, delay worry to your next designated worry time.

    *   Notice. (*Oh, there is a worry.*)

    *   Validate. (*I can absolutely worry about this.*)

    *   Delay. (*And, I have set aside time to do so. I will worry about this at 5:15 this evening. Or: And, I have already done so today. I will have another chance tomorrow.*)

    *   Refocus your attention on something else.

The word that best describes what my mind does when I am in bed awake is:

_____   Worries (harasses me with concerns about the future)

_____   Reminisces (thinks fondly about the past)

_____   Problem-solves (defines a problem; generates and considers potential solutions)

_____   Plans (generates "To Do" lists; rehearses a presentation; thinks about what needs to be packed for a trip)

_____   Fantasizes (imagines desired future scenarios)

_____   Races (lots of thoughts, moving quickly)

_____   Ruminates (reviews the past again and again)

_____   Other: _____

My designated time to do this type of thinking (for example: "11 a.m.," "Before lunch," "After dinner," "Just before kids come home," "Variable—will put in day-timer Sunday night for the next week"):

How long I will give my mind to think this way (for example, "ten minutes"):

Strategies for remembering my designated time (for example: "Set alarm," "Put note in lunch bag"):

Strategies for getting out of my head at the end of my designated time (for example: "Set timer," "Mindful breathing," "Have lunch with others," "Know what I am going to do next"):

What I will tell myself if I notice myself thinking this way outside of my designated time:

Am I willing to try this strategy for at least one or two weeks?

How to Evaluate Your Progress and When to Consider a Different Strategy

We love the delighted surprise in our client's voices when, after trying DWT for a week or two, they say, "It really works!" If DWT is helping you, you will know it. Most likely you will notice that you can more easily let go of worries (or other thought processes) outside of your designated time, including when you would rather be sleeping. You may have the experience of running out of things to think about during your designated time. Or you may recognize that you worry about the same things each and every day. These experiences often lead to "aha" moments.

For example, one client said, "I realized that if I can't even fill ten minutes, I can't possibly have enough to worry about to keep me up all night!" Others realize that their active minds are not really serving up anything new. This recognition helps them detach and quiet their minds when it is time to sleep. For example, they respond to their worry thoughts by saying to themselves, *Yes, I can think about this, but there's really nothing new here. I might as well wait until my next designated time.*

If you do not think you are benefiting from DWT, there are two common culprits to consider. First, is it not working because you are not doing it? Some people simply will not try DWT at all. Others try to get away with delaying the worry forever, without ever having regular worry sessions. If you have not been willing to do both steps of DWT, why not? Do you think it will not be helpful to you? You may be right if you are not a worrier *and* your mind is not particularly active during your sleep window. If this is the case, we agree that you would be better served putting your time and energy into other strategies. On the other hand, if you are a worrier *or* if your mind is active when you want to be sleeping, then we encourage you to work toward increased willingness to try DWT. As we said earlier, we have found DWT to be an incredibly useful strategy for so many of our clients, even those who were skeptical or scared when we first introduced it. How to increase your willingness depends on what the blocks are. You may want to revisit the concept of willingness (chapter 4), use cognitive restructuring (chapter 10) to work through thoughts that are getting in the way, or problem-solve practical obstacles like not having the privacy or time you need.

The second common culprit is rumination. As we already have explained, when people ruminate about the past, they feel worse. If you are feeling worse after trying DWT, ask yourself whether your mind is like a "broken record" during your designated time. Use the tips we provided above to shift from ruminating about the past to projecting into the future. Then, reevaluate the effect of DWT.

Your Next Step

If DWT has been helpful, continue to use this tool in addition to working your behavioral sleep program. Then, once you have been following your behavioral program for at least six to eight weeks, you are welcome to skip to chapter 13 to evaluate your progress. Or you may want to learn additional cognitive strategies to help you stop the insomnia spiral.

In the next chapter we provide additional tools for quieting your mind. You may choose to use these strategies instead of DWT, or in addition to it. Mindfulness in particular complements the delay part of DWT, so we especially encourage you to read the next chapter if you have a hard time shifting your focus away from your worries, even with the promise that you soon will allow your mind to worry, worry, worry.

Or perhaps practicing DWT made you aware of patterns of negative thinking, such as always predicting the worst possible outcome. If this is the case and you have not yet worked through chapter 10, this may be a good time to learn how to work with the content of your thoughts using cognitive restructuring.

Chapter 12

Accepting Your Thoughts (Mindfulness and Cognitive Defusion)

*T*his chapter is about using acceptance-based cognitive tools to optimize your personalized sleep plan. Developing and implementing a personalized sleep program can be very challenging. You are tired of being tired and you want an immediate solution. Unfortunately, CBT-I programs are not geared toward immediate relief. You must tolerate additional discomfort before you see results. You must also change your current habits and patterns. You must convince your already frustrated mind to choose to do something different. You are required to complete worksheets and redesign your daytime and nighttime rituals.

Acceptance-based tools can help you to manage all of these challenges.

As the name implies, the basic premise is that there is benefit to being open and accepting of all of your experiences, including your thoughts. This is a paradigm shift, because our natural response to uncomfortable thoughts is to judge them, evaluate them, and react to them. Thus, the focus of acceptance-based cognitive skills is to train your mind to respond to your thoughts in a different way. We have found that these skills are complementary to the traditional cognitive skills that are taught in CBT-I.

Poor sleepers typically have a hard time turning off the "mind chatter" (Lundh & Hindmarsh, 2002). Busy brains interfere with falling asleep and staying asleep. You may experience this as being "tired but wired." In fact, people with insomnia have more of this disruptive mental activity than healthy sleepers (Nofzinger et al., 2004). Additionally, poor sleepers worry more and work harder at trying to control their thoughts than healthy sleepers (Harvey, 2001). Acceptance-based tools address all of these challenges.

Who Should Use Mindfulness and Cognitive Defusion?

The acceptance-based tools of mindfulness training and cognitive defusion can help you to manage your busy, active mind. This is especially helpful when you are trying to sleep. It is also useful for decreasing your overall arousal during the day. Finally, these strategies can help you relate differently to thoughts that interfere with your willingness to change your sleep-related behaviors. Here are some clues that these acceptance-based tools will likely be useful for you:

- You have racing thoughts at bedtime or during the night.

- You have repetitive thoughts that cycle like a tape through your mind.

- You get increasingly frustrated and discouraged when you are not sleeping.

- You have intrusive and anxiety-provoking thoughts about your sleep (at any time of day).

- Stressful thoughts about other areas of your life show up at bedtime or during the night.

- You believe that you are not capable of making a behavioral change you think would be helpful.

- You believe that behavioral strategies will not help your insomnia.

- You are using designated worry time and have trouble delaying your worry.

Mental Fitness

You can use acceptance-based skills with all thoughts. These skills help us remember that thoughts are not facts. Thoughts are just thoughts; they may be true or false or something in between. Acceptance is not about liking or wanting particular thoughts. It is about allowing thoughts to be present *without the thoughts influencing your choices* in unhelpful ways. "Unhelpful" refers to anything that does not support your values and goals.

It can be helpful to think of acceptance-based skills as skills to improve your mental fitness. Fitness is your general state of health and well-being. Fitness provides the strength and endurance you need to achieve your goals. You can improve your physical fitness skills through cardiovascular exercise, weight-training, and stretching or yoga. Each of these practices contributes to your body's ability to do the physical things you care about. Think back to our discussion about skiing trees and you will probably agree with us that your capacity to be successful is likely to be greater if you have been strengthening and stretching your body in preparation.

Mental fitness is just like physical fitness. It then follows that your capacity to be successful with a challenging and often uncomfortable sleep program is likely to be greater if you have been strengthening and stretching your mind in preparation. Mental fitness skills will help you tip your scale back toward the side of restorative sleep. These skills will help you quiet your busy mind. They will also help you stick with your sleep program.

Mental Fitness and Sleep

There are countless mental fitness skills. Willingness is an example of a mental fitness skill because it encourages your mind to be open, or accepting, of your experiences. We covered this in chapter 4 because we so often find it helpful to work on this early in treatment.

In this chapter we are going to focus on the two additional mental fitness skills we have found to be most relevant to sleep. They are mindfulness and cognitive defusion. Poor sleepers who practice these types of skills have been able to increase their ability to have restful and restorative sleep (Ong & Sholtes, 2010). Mindfulness and cognitive defusion skills can be practiced anywhere at any time. You can do them in a more formal setting with props such as pillows and guided recordings, or you can do them informally with nothing but your mind and your breath. This book contains guided recordings to assist you in practicing these skills.

Mindfulness

Mindfulness is intentional focus on the here and now. It is when you are "full of mind." It refers to any time you deliberately choose to pay attention to what is happening in this moment. Let's try an example. Set a timer for thirty seconds. Ask yourself to use those thirty seconds to pay close attention to the sounds around you. This can be done with eyes open or closed and with your body in any comfortable position. Just try your best to intentionally focus on the sounds around you. Once the time has passed, ask yourself the following questions.

1. What did I hear?

2. Did the sounds change over the thirty seconds?

3. Did I notice any new or different sounds?

4. Did I have any opinions or thoughts during this time?

5. Did my attention wander while I was trying to focus on listening to sounds? If yes, where did my mind go?

This is an example of mindfulness training. You engaged in a deliberate and focused exercise to be fully in this moment. In this exercise, you used one of your five senses to guide your focus. You identified the ways your focus shifted (or not). You also noticed what, if any, thoughts showed up. There is no need to assess how well you did this mindful exercise because there is really no correct way of practicing mindfulness. It just takes a willingness to pay attention to your attention. Studies have shown that a daily mindfulness practice (with a cumulative total of approximately thirty minutes) can influence our brains in as little as eight weeks (Hölzel et al., 2011).

Mindfulness is not about achieving a state of happiness or contentment or a blank mind. Oftentimes the information we receive when we pay attention to the present moment is unpleasant or painful. Mindfulness is about using your focus and your awareness to be as open as possible to what you are experiencing right here, right now. Mindfulness is about being present with whatever thoughts, feelings, and sensations you experience. Through mindfulness training you can improve your ability to notice whatever shows up, without necessarily having to act on it. This can help you stay on track with your goals. For example, mindfulness can be helpful when you notice your anxious thoughts about your sleep program. You can be mindful of these thoughts *and* proceed with the program anyway because it is consistent with your goal of improving your sleep.

When you hear the term "mindfulness" you may also think of meditation. There is a vast amount of information on the similarities and dissimilarities of these two concepts. For our purposes, we will use the term "mindfulness" to refer to the intentional practice of paying attention to this moment. We will use the term "meditation" to refer to a specific type of "formal" mindfulness practice. However, we don't want you to worry too much about these labels. No matter what you call it, strengthening your ability to focus and pay attention, on purpose, is tremendously helpful with sleep. This is because you are teaching your mind to have contact with the present moment. This will allow you to quiet your mind if an active mind is keeping you awake. It also will allow you to notice anxiety- or arousal-provoking thoughts and respond to them with equanimity.

Mindfulness Exercises

There are many opinions about how to practice mindfulness. Many mindfulness exercises use the breath as an anchor, but mindfulness does not always have to involve your breath. The most important guideline that we know of is this: just try something! Mindfulness is not a skill you can gain by reading about it or watching a video. You have to do it. Here are some helpful ideas on how to get started.

Five senses. Your five senses are a priceless resource. They are with you whenever you need them. Use them to pay attention. Start with thirty seconds at a time. Pick one of your senses and repeat the exercise we described in the beginning of this section. Notice what you hear, smell, taste, touch, or see. Pay attention to your attention. Be prepared to lose focus; when you do, gently encourage your mind to return to the sense on which you are focusing.

Ordinary or automatic tasks. Your boring or tedious tasks can become an invaluable resource! Tasks such as brushing your teeth, folding laundry, or washing dishes often encourage daydreaming and minimal focus. Engage in one of these activities with the goal of paying attention only to the task. Let's use brushing your teeth as an example. You may notice how the tube of toothpaste feels in your hand, and how your fingers know just how much pressure to use to get the paste onto your brush. Pay attention to your arm lifting your toothbrush to your mouth, and how your lips know just when to part. Notice where in your mouth you start to brush, and the sensations of the brush and toothpaste on your teeth and gums. Pay attention to your attention. Be prepared to lose focus; when you do, gently direct your attention back to the task.

Music. Choose a song you know and love. Listen to it five times in a row. Each time you listen, pick a specific instrument (for example, drums, vocals, or guitar) to focus on. Listen and focus on this instrument only. Pay attention to your attention. Be prepared to lose focus; when you do, gently encourage your mind to return to the instrument. Now choose a song that is unfamiliar to you. Repeat the exercise.

Breath. Like your senses, your breath can be counted on to be there. Always. You can always return to your breath and find it waiting there for you. Start with thirty seconds. Pay attention to your breath. Notice each inhale and each exhale. There is no need to change your breath, nor is there any need to keep it the same. Simply notice each breath, as it is. Pay attention to your attention. Be prepared to lose focus; when you do, gently direct your attention back to your breath.

If you find this thirty-second practice useful, you might try practicing longer—five minutes, or better yet, ten. You can use the guided audio files that are available at the website for this book: http://www.newharbinger.com/33438.

Summary of Mindfulness Exercises

Mindfulness is a practice. It is a skill that develops over time. Mindfulness training creates strength and flexibility. It is one way to improve mental fitness. Optimal practice involves daily commitment. Three minutes every day is more valuable than two hours once a week. Mindfulness can be that accessible.

Cognitive Defusion

Cognitive defusion, our second mental fitness tool, comes from acceptance and commitment therapy (ACT). It is derived from the understanding that we can get tangled up and lost in our thoughts. We can literally get "fused" with thoughts. We lose sight of ourselves. We also lose sight of other, often helpful, information. Think about the zoom lens on a camera. When you zoom in, the focus is on one small part of the picture. Your zoom lens screens out all the other information. Now imagine that your eye becomes fused with the lens itself. You are no longer a person looking through a lens. You are the lens. You have no separation between you as a person and you as that lens. That is fusion.

Please note that fusion is not "bad." Fusion can be helpful in certain situations. When you are driving in traffic it is crucial to pay attention. You want all of your thoughts and awareness to zoom in on your driving. You want to ignore the distractions around you, such as the radio or your phone. In sleep-related situations, however, fusion is often unhelpful. When you are trying to fall asleep, it can be problematic to zoom in on the experience. The zoom lens amplifies your fears. When you get fused to your thoughts in these moments, you end up in the insomnia spiral.

Cognitive defusion is a skill that helps you to step back from the thoughts your mind is generating. In defusion, we are less interested in whether the statements are true, and more interested in how to shift to a wide-angle lens. This is about the relationship between you and your thoughts. When you "defuse" yourself from the content of your mind, you help yourself, and your mind, to be more objective and less reactive.

Cognitive Defusion Exercises

There are many ways to practice cognitive defusion. As with mindfulness, the key is to *engage* in experiential exercises. Thinking and reading about defusion is helpful, but will not directly improve your mental fitness. Here are some helpful ideas on how to get started.

Name it to tame it. Think of one or two of your most distressing thoughts about sleep. Say them to yourself several times. Now write them down on a piece of paper. Take the paper and put it on the floor in front of you, about two feet away. Read these thoughts to yourself. Now read them again while walking around the piece of paper in a circle. Keep these thoughts in your head as you turn your back to the paper.

What did you notice? You may have had a thought like, *Oh there is that thought again, it's like a broken record.* Or you may have said to yourself, *Here I am, standing over these thoughts and I wonder why I am doing this.* No matter what you thought, it is likely that you got a sense of you as a person, separate from these thoughts. You are you, and those words on the piece of paper are your thoughts. *You are not your thoughts.* No matter what the content of your thoughts are, you are here in this moment noticing thoughts. You have these thoughts but they do not have you. That is cognitive defusion.

Television ticker. Think of the television programs, such as the news, sports channels, and weather stations, that provide ongoing information. The television ticker consists of a constant stream of words going across the bottom of the screen. The information at the bottom of the screen just keeps showing up. Sometimes it is new information; other times it is old information being repeated. Oftentimes there is additional programming going on simultaneously.

Now imagine that your thoughts are the content of this ticker line at the bottom of the screen. You are the person watching this information move across the screen. Sometimes it is new information. Frequently, it just repeats a story. When you notice that you are here and your thoughts are there (on the screen), you are practicing cognitive defusion.

Play with the "packaging." Another way to defuse from thoughts is to play around with their form. There are lots of ways to do this.

- Sing your thoughts! Make them sound like opera, or set them to the tune of a familiar song or jingle.

- Say your thoughts in a funny but familiar voice, such as that of Donald Duck.

- Type out a thought on your computer screen. Copy it multiple times, and put each repetition in a different font size and style.

- All of these exercises can help you remember that thoughts are just thoughts.

Thank you, mind. Cognitive defusion can be as simple as saying "Thank you" to your mind. Try it out the next time your mind gives you a challenging thought about sleep.

Your mind: "I am never going to fall asleep."

You: "Thanks, mind."

Your mind: "This book won't be able to help me."

You: "Thanks, mind."

Make sure your tone is one of compassion and kindness. Your response should be one of sincerity, not sarcasm. You may not like what your mind is telling you, but you can still thank it. Your mind is only doing what it is designed to do. Minds are designed to generate thoughts, feelings, urges, sensations, and memories at a staggering rate. Your mind also reminds you that you are only doing what you are designed to do. You are designed to notice all of this information. You are designed to let this information support, but not dominate you.

More choices. There are other exercises you can use to practice defusion skills, of course. For example, you could imagine yourself at a parade with your thoughts on the signs that people in the procession are carrying, and just watch those thoughts go by. We have made audio versions to guide you in a couple of defusion exercises; visit http://www.newharbinger.com/33438 to try them.

Example: George's Use of Mindfulness and Defusion

We are going to use George, whom we introduced in chapter 3, to illustrate these skills. George is a self-employed businessman and father of three children. His sleep problems started after the birth of his third child. His current difficulties include trouble falling asleep and waking too early in the morning (around 3 a.m.). He is fatigued during the day, concerned about his job productivity, and anxious about how to fix his sleep problems.

George has an active and busy mind. His thoughts are repetitive and racing during the day and during the night.

As part of his sleep program, George starts practicing mindfulness exercises during the daytime. Each day he does at least one routine task mindfully, such as brushing his teeth, lathering on his shaving cream, or kissing his children good-bye. At the office he practices slowing down: after hanging up the phone he takes three mindful breaths before he places his next phone call; and he walks mindfully when going from his office to the conference room or bathroom.

After about a week of practicing being mindful in his daily life, George starts to set aside five or ten minutes for a "formal" mindfulness exercise. Sometimes he uses one of the guided recordings; other times he practices in silence. He usually does this in the evening, after the children have gone to bed. Sometimes the mindfulness exercise has a calming effect. Other times it makes him even more aware of painful emotions and sensations. George reminds himself that the goal is not to feel a certain way. The goal is to be open to all feelings.

George continues to have a busy mind at night. His daytime mindfulness practice helps: when he is lying in bed, he is better able to let go of his thoughts and focus instead on his breath. Sometimes. He decides to add cognitive defusion skills to further untangle himself from his thoughts. His go-to method is to picture his thoughts on the ticker at the bottom of a television screen, though he sometimes places his thoughts on pickets carried by people in a parade, or on leaves floating down a stream.

With a lot of practice and a big dose of willingness, George is better able to step back from his overactive mind and drop into the present moment. He can still enjoy a fast-paced mind when it serves him well during the day. But he can also take brief breaks during the day and feel less frenetic. And he is better able to disengage from his thoughts when he would rather be sleeping.

How Mindfulness and Cognitive Defusion Go Awry

There are two common challenges with mindfulness and cognitive defusion. The first is using acceptance skills with a change agenda. An example of this is using mindfulness or cognitive defusion during the night specifically to help you fall asleep. The trap has been set; you are using your skills to change your situation. This is a trap because the goal of these skills is not to change your situation, but to increase your acceptance of the situation.

Mental fitness skills work best when your intention is to accept whatever is happening as it is, without judgment and without expectation of it being different. In these moments, it is important to remind yourself that you are using mental fitness skills to accept that you are awake, when you would rather be asleep.

The second challenge is knowing when and where to practice mindfulness and cognitive defusion. Of course you will be most motivated to try these skills when you are struggling with falling asleep! This is akin to trying to improve your cardiovascular fitness in the midst of a race. Fitness skills need to be honed in advance. They require time and consistency to build your strength and stamina. It is recommended that you first practice mindfulness and cognitive defusion during the daytime hours (or when you are in your wake cycle). After you have established proficiency during your wake cycle, you then can utilize these skills during your sleep cycle.

Common Obstacles (and Possible Solutions)

"I do not have time."

Use some of the mindfulness and defusion exercises with this statement. What happens when you step back from this thought? In the few moments it took to work with this thought, you engaged in the very skills you do not have time for! It is as simple and straightforward as that.

"It is too spiritual (or too religious, or too unscientific)."

Although mindfulness has a long tradition in Buddhism and Hinduism, it also can be practiced in a nonreligious, nonspiritual fashion. Over the past several decades, researchers such as Jon Kabat-Zinn and Jeffrey Brantley have applied mindfulness to the treatment of a number of ailments. Mindfulness has gained strong scientific support in our Western world. It is now widely recognized as a useful intervention for both medical and psychiatric issues. Cognitive defusion also is scientifically based. It was largely developed in the psychology laboratory of Steven Hayes. Consider checking out these researchers' publications to learn more about the science of mindfulness and cognitive defusion.

"It is just a popular trend right now."

Mindfulness and cognitive defusion are certainly popular right now. For good reason. The studies are consistently and significantly showing the benefits. Even when the trend moves on to something else, you can be sure the benefits will still be here.

"When I try it, I get really uncomfortable." Or: "When I try it, I get really emotional."

Yes, mental fitness can be hard to practice. These skills are, at times, uncomfortable. Remember the value of discomfort. Establish some personal guidelines for what is outside your comfort zone but not pushing you into your danger zone. When you are just outside your comfort zone, give yourself reassurance and praise. If you see yourself headed to your danger zone, take a break.

"It does not help me to fall asleep."

These skills were not developed to help you fall asleep. They were designed to help you accept what is going on, at any given time. You happen to be caught in the spiral of insomnia. These skills will help you interrupt that spiral by allowing you to relate differently to your thoughts. By accepting instead of struggling, and by stepping back from your thoughts, you can decrease your physiological arousal. This will help your body be more primed for sleep, but it will not help you to control your sleep.

Also, these skills will help you to follow through with your program. When your mind serves up obstacles to doing stimulus control or sleep restriction fully, or to making uncomfortable behavioral changes, you can use mindfulness and defusion to deftly navigate these obstacles. You can thank your mind, and then continue to do what we know will help you sleep better in the long term.

"I do not like practicing mental fitness. Do I have to do it?"

No. You do not have to do anything you do not want to do. However, consider whether there is value in trying it anyway. You do not have to like it to find benefit.

Your Mindfulness and Cognitive Defusion Plan

Use worksheet 12.1 to record your practice of mindfulness and cognitive defusion. Spend some time considering what types of exercises you would like to use. Set up a time that you will practice these skills. Use reminders, such as Post-it notes or alarms on your phone, to support your plan. Check out the audio recordings that accompany this book (available at www.newharbinger.com/33438) to see if any of these will provide useful guidance.

WORKSHEET 12.1: Your Mindfulness and Cognitive Defusion Plan

Exercises I am interested in trying include:

_____   Mindfulness using five senses

_____   Mindfulness of an ordinary daily task

_____   Mindfulness of music

_____   Mindfulness of breath

_____   Name it to tame it defusion exercise

_____   Defuse from my thoughts by seeing them go by on a television ticker (or similar imagery)

_____   Defuse from my thoughts by singing them, saying them in a funny voice, or typing them in different fonts

_____   Defuse from my thoughts by thanking my mind

_____   Guided exercises (audio files available with this book or from other sources)

_____   Other: _____

My goal is to practice _____ times a week, for at least _____ minutes.

Preparations to make ahead of time (for example, download guided exercises, research local mindfulness groups):

Strategies for remembering to practice (for example, schedule time on calendar, set alert on phone):

My Practice Log

Date	Exercise	Duration	Notes

What to Expect

You can expect a nonlinear learning curve with mindfulness and cognitive defusion: two steps forward, one step back. Some days you will find it easier to be mindful of the present moment and defused from your thoughts than on other days. You will notice more improvement if you practice on a daily basis. These skills require consistency and repetition. As your mental fitness increases, you will notice that you are less reactive to your busy mind. You will be able to quiet a busy mind while lying in bed. You will be able to choose a focus such as your breath and keep returning to this focus. Your capacity to hold this focus will increase. Your capacity to recognize when your focus has strayed, and to bring it back, will increase. Mindfulness training can help you become more aware of your thoughts, which is the first step in cognitive restructuring. With designated worry time, mindfulness training can help you more quickly notice when your mind is worrying. Then, when you decide to delay worry to your next DWT, you can use mindfulness to help you shift your attention to the present moment (or whatever you want to focus on). Similarly, you can use the skill of cognitive defusion to say to yourself, *Oh, there's worry. Thanks, mind, but I will worry later!* These acceptance-based skills can optimize your ability to work on these change-based cognitive skills.

How to Evaluate Your Progress

We have made the point that with mindfulness practice you are not trying to achieve any one particular outcome, such as a blank mind or calm state. Mindfulness is meant to be a "nonstriving" practice. How, then, can you determine whether or not it is "working"? Use effectiveness as your compass.

Although you may not feel relaxed each time you practice mindfulness, practicing regularly can certainly make you feel more centered or calm throughout the day. Are you noticing any decrease in the type of anxious arousal that may be feeding your insomnia spiral? Are you able to use what you have learned in your daytime mindfulness practice to quiet your mind when you are in bed?

Is your practice with cognitive defusion strategies helping you step back from your thoughts? For example, can you notice thoughts like *I am so tired, I have to stay in bed longer,* but then choose not to act on them? Are you taking less seriously all the catastrophic thoughts about your sleep that your mind serves up? If your mind is busy at bedtime or during a middle-of-the-night awakening (when cognitive restructuring may be too arousing), are you able to use defusion strategies to disengage?

Your Next Step

Look back at the treatment plan you developed using worksheet 5.1. Are you already making use of all of the strategies you selected? Have you been doing your core behavioral treatment for at least six to eight weeks? If so, you are ready for part 4 of this book, which will help you evaluate your progress, change your plan if you need to, and maintain any gains you have made.

Otherwise, continue to work your program. You may want to linger here, focusing on the strategies you already are using. Or you may want to continue to add to your toolbox with the cognitive or behavioral strategies you are not yet using. Of course, continue to track your progress using your sleep log and your Sleep Log Summary worksheet.

Summary of Part 3

COGNITIVE STRATEGIES

Our thoughts play a big role in our lives. Thoughts provide a constant stream of information, and they have the capacity to both promote and interfere with sleep. The cognitive strategies we just reviewed are an essential part of your sleep program. These skills will help you address the perpetuating factors that tip your sleep scale toward insomnia. They will help you relate to your thoughts differently, which will, in itself, promote restorative sleep. These skills will also increase your ability to stick with your sleep program. Are you willing to bring this component into your personalized treatment plan?

Part 4

Reviewing Your Progress and Maintaining Your Gains

Chapter 13

How Effective Is Your Program?

We expect this chapter to be most useful to you after six to eight weeks of actively working your integrated treatment program (not including the initial weeks in which you collected data and formed your treatment plan). If you are still in the thick of treatment, return to this chapter later. If you have been working a behavioral program (stimulus control, sleep restriction, or the combination) for at least six to eight weeks, then it is time to take stock. After you take stock, we will help you figure out your next steps.

Taking Stock

In chapter 1 we emphasized the importance of using data—not just your memory or general sense of things—to track your sleep. Hopefully you have been keeping a sleep log and completing the Sleep Log Summary worksheet throughout your treatment program. If you have not been, go ahead and collect some data for a week or two.

How Are You Sleeping?

Use the Sleep Log Summary from chapter 5 (worksheet 5.2 or 5.3) to see how you are sleeping now compared with before your treatment program. The following list describes some elements you likely will be interested in. Your particular flavor of insomnia coming into this treatment will dictate which of these variables are the most useful measures of progress. You can look at the goals you set on worksheet 5.1 to remind yourself of the changes you were hoping for.

Total sleep time (TST). Take a look at the amount of sleep you are getting each night. Is your TST close to the amount of sleep your body needs? Or do you consider yourself to be sleep deprived on a regular basis? If you are not getting enough sleep, then it is worth comparing your current TST to your pretreatment TST. Is it trending in the right direction, or has it not improved at all?

If you are hitting your body's target, that is great! And it really does not matter if you are getting more sleep than before treatment. Perhaps you were getting enough sleep before treatment, and you have been working toward having better quality sleep, rather than more sleep. Or maybe before treatment you had some "good" nights (for example, eight and a half hours TST) and some "bad" nights (for example, three hours TST), which balanced out to an acceptable average TST (for example, seven hours). If you now are getting a steady seven hours each night, you likely are feeling much better even though there has been no change in your average TST.

Hours in bed and sleep efficiency (SE). How many hours are you spending in bed? What proportion of that time is spent asleep? Is this different than before the treatment?

This is an area in which we frequently see a lot of improvement. If you are like many of our clients, you were giving sleep a lot of room, and it was occupying only a portion of that space. For example, you may have been setting aside nine hours of sleep opportunity, and getting six hours of sleep. That means you had three unused hours that were dedicated to sleep. Which means you had three fewer hours to live your life. It may be helpful to do a little extra arithmetic to highlight any gains you made: subtract your average hours in bed from twenty-four to see how many hours you are up and about!

We would not expect to see improved SE if you had adapted to your insomnia by spending less time in bed. That is, some people say that they do not bother going to bed until much later than their preferred bedtime, because they know they will not sleep anyway. Others say that when they wake up at 3 a.m. they simply get up and start their day. If this sounds like you, then an increase in time in bed, coupled with an increase in TST, will be a better measure of progress than a change in SE.

Sleep onset latency (SOL). How long is it between "lights out" and when you fall asleep? If it is taking you less than twenty minutes to fall asleep, we consider this to be in the normal range. If your SOL was normal before your treatment program, then you may not see a change on this measure. On the other hand, if you were having trouble falling asleep in the beginning of the night, then we want to see this number go down over the course of treatment.

Awakenings. How many times during the night do you wake up? If you wake once or twice a night and can quickly fall back to sleep, this is completely normal. In fact, some studies suggest that the typical person wakes up for at least thirty seconds six times a night (Smith et al., 2003)! Therefore, we would not necessarily expect treatment to rid you of all awakenings. We also would not expect CBT-I to decrease awakenings caused by a child or bed partner, or by a medical condition (such as an enlarged prostate that makes you have to urinate frequently). If, on the other hand, you were waking multiple times a night without explanation, then we would hope to be seeing fewer awakenings.

Wake after sleep onset (WASO). For how many minutes are you awake in the middle of the night (after you first fall asleep, but before your final awakening)? Even if you only wake up once, this can be a huge disruption if you are awake for a long time. If you had more than twenty minutes of WASO before treatment, we hope your treatment program reduced this to less than ten minutes.

How Do You Feel During the Day?

Now let's shift our focus from how you are sleeping at night to how you feel and function during your waking hours. Here are the questions we asked you in chapter 1. Answer these questions again, without peeking at your previous responses.

TABLE 13.1: What Insomnia Is Costing Me Now

Think about how you feel and behave the day after a poor night's sleep. Also think about the overall, cumulative effect of your ongoing sleep problems. Now look at this list of common daytime consequences of insomnia.

Circle the number of days in a typical week you experience each consequence *because of sleep disturbance.*

For any items you scored 1 or more, rate how much this affects you:

0 = No big deal; I barely even noticed or thought about it until you asked.

1 = Mild impact/somewhat distressing.

2 = Moderate impact/quite distressing.

3 = Significant impact/extremely distressing.

For example, if you are late to work three times a week, this may not be a problem at all because you have lots of flexibility and you do not mind shifting your work hours (0); or it may cause some personal frustration but no real problems at work or with your after-work plans (1); or it may cause problems with your boss/coworkers/employees/clients, or with other activities because you have to make up the time (2); or it may get you fired or make you lose business (3).

Because of insomnia I...	# Days in a Typical Week								Impact (0–3)
...am late to work, school, or other activities.	0	1	2	3	4	5	6	7	
...stay home from work or school, or cancel professional obligations.	0	1	2	3	4	5	6	7	
...perform below expectations or am less productive.	0	1	2	3	4	5	6	7	
...socialize less.	0	1	2	3	4	5	6	7	
...exercise less.	0	1	2	3	4	5	6	7	
...skip evening activities because I am too tired.	0	1	2	3	4	5	6	7	
...skip evening activities because I am worried they will disrupt my sleep.	0	1	2	3	4	5	6	7	
...have a harder time remembering things.	0	1	2	3	4	5	6	7	
...have a harder time focusing or concentrating.	0	1	2	3	4	5	6	7	
...am irritable with other people.	0	1	2	3	4	5	6	7	
...am more sad, tearful, or anxious.	0	1	2	3	4	5	6	7	
...worry about sleep during the day.	0	1	2	3	4	5	6	7	
...feel anxious about how I will sleep that night.	0	1	2	3	4	5	6	7	
...think about terrible things that may happen because of my insomnia (for example, impact on health, performance, relationships).	0	1	2	3	4	5	6	7	
...fall asleep at inopportune times (for example, during meetings or classes, or while watching movies).	0	1	2	3	4	5	6	7	
...am too tired to drive safely.	0	1	2	3	4	5	6	7	
...feel physically uncomfortable (for example, burning eyes or headaches).	0	1	2	3	4	5	6	7	

Now look back at your earlier responses. What has changed? What has stayed the same? Overall, is insomnia costing you less? If so, how much less? Or is insomnia costing you even more? Most often, insomnia is costing people less at this point in treatment. However, sometimes it is costing them more because of the time and effort they are putting into treatment. If this is true for you, know that this increased cost likely will not last much longer.

You also may want to look at your average fatigue rating if you completed this on the Expanded Sleep Log Summary. Has this changed over time? If you are getting more sleep or your sleep is more consolidated, then you may feel better rested. It is also possible that you had an increase in fatigue or sleepiness after starting stimulus control or sleep restriction therapy. If so, we would expect this to be getting better after six to eight weeks of continuous treatment.

Have You Found Your Sweet Spot?

From the very beginning of this book, we have encouraged you to *commit fully* to your treatment program, in order to give it the best chance of working. This probably required you to be willing to do things that were uncomfortable. We also have encouraged you to be *flexible*: we have asked you to use *effectiveness* rather than rigid rules to guide your treatment. This has included shifting your focus from trying to sleep tonight to a longer-term goal of consistent, reliable sleep. Indeed, we have even asked you to be willing to not sleep tonight, in order to decrease your struggle.

Have you found your sweet spot? Are you being rigid enough that you are actually doing the treatment as prescribed, but not so rigid that you are feeding the insomnia spiral with increased anxiety or arousal? Let's take a look at each part of this equation.

How Closely Have You Followed Your Treatment Program?

It is time to take a really honest look at how closely you have followed your treatment program. You may want to look back at worksheet 5.1 to remind yourself which strategies you selected when you put together your individualized treatment plan. Then, assess your follow-through using these steps:

Step 1: Review the basic instructions of each treatment strategy you used.

Step 2: Look at your sleep logs and relevant worksheets to see how closely you followed the instructions.

Here are some examples of what you might ask yourself for each treatment component. If you can answer yes to all of the questions, you did an amazing job using the strategy as it is meant to be used!

Stimulus control therapy. Does my sleep log show that I was in bed awake for no more than twenty minutes at a time? Is "lights out" the same time as when I got "into bed," such that I did not do other things in bed? Did I do all of my sleeping in bed? Did I get up at the same time each day (and not go back to bed or to sleep), regardless of how much sleep I got? Did I have no daytime naps?

Sleep restriction therapy. Did I limit my time in bed to the amount of sleep I was averaging before treatment (or to five hours if I was averaging less than that)? Did I have a consistent sleep schedule? Did I have no daytime naps? Did I increase my time in bed by fifteen minutes at a time, and no more than once per week? Did I wait until my sleep efficiency was 90% before increasing my time in bed?

Sleep hygiene. Looking at the goals I set in step 2 of worksheet 9.1, did I regularly do what I set out to do? (For example: On how many nights did I engage in my wind-down routine? On how many mornings did I wake "briskly" and rise when I first awoke?)

Cognitive restructuring. Did I pay attention to my thoughts each day? Did I complete thought records for thoughts that were contributing to my insomnia spiral? Did I actually write stuff down, and not "just think about it"? As I identified and challenged distorted or unhelpful thoughts, was I also willing to have those thoughts come into my mind (or did I try to "control" my thoughts such that cognitive restructuring added to my struggle)?

Designated worry time. Did I set aside time during the day and indulge my mind in the type of thinking (worrying, reminiscing, problem-solving, planning, fantasizing, racing) that interferes with sleep? Did I stay on task so that my mind could become satiated? (For example, if you worry at night, did you only worry during DWT, and not veer off into problem-solving?) Did I make sure *not* to *ruminate* during my designated time? If my mind was busy when I wanted to be sleeping, did I remind myself that I could think this way, but I would do so at my next designated time?

Mindfulness. Did I practice regularly (five to seven days per week)? Did I try a variety of mindfulness training exercises?

Cognitive defusion. Did I practice regularly (five to seven days per week)? Did I try a variety of defusion exercises?

Why are we encouraging you to take such a close look? Clients often tell us that they did things when they did not, or did not do them fully. For example, people say that they did stimulus control, and their sleep logs show that they were in bed awake for an hour. We are not interested in giving you a poor grade or correcting you with a red pen. We *do* want you to have accurate information about what you have tried. As you will see, this is essential as you plan your next steps (below) and develop a plan to help you maintain any gains you have made (chapter 14).

There is another reason we want you to have accurate information about what you have and have not tried. When people think they have done what was advised, and they are not sleeping better, this feeds into hopelessness and despair. It adds to cognitive distortions such as *Nothing is going to help*. If, instead, you realize that you have not implemented the treatment fully, you may shift your thinking to something like: *I took a low dose of sleep restriction. Maybe if I do it more fully it will work for me*. Now, instead of giving up, you may redouble your effort and tackle whatever roadblocks got in the way of doing the treatment fully.

Have You Used Effectiveness as Your Compass?

In chapter 4 we asked you to think about how you struggle with sleep. Revisit the questions we posed there. Have you been applying any of the components of your treatment program in such a rigid fashion that this has added to your struggle? For example, if your target bedtime in your behavioral program is 10:30, did you become so concerned about varying from this that you gave up an important social engagement? Or were you able to be more flexible and stay out late? Did you find the sweet spot, by going to bed later (demonstrating flexibility) but still getting up at your consistent wake time (sticking with the program)? Finally, did you use this experience to collect data and see what happened when you varied your sleep schedule, so that you can make an informed decision if you are again confronted with this challenge?

The Next Leg of Your Adventure

What you do next will depend on a combination of how much progress you have made toward your goal and how closely you have been following the guidelines of the treatment strategies you have been using. Figure 13.1 provides a visual depiction of the roadmap we use to help people decide on their next step.

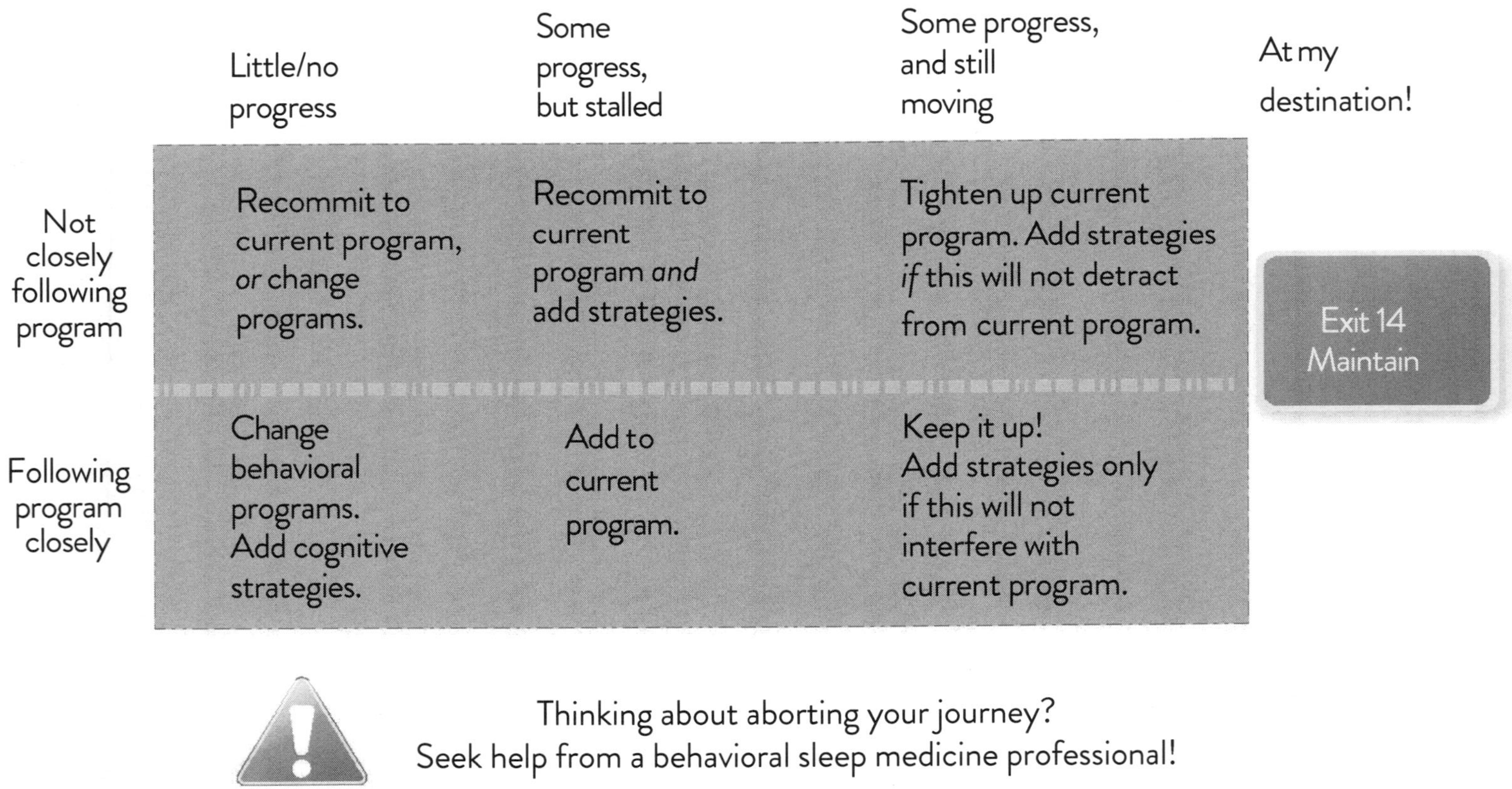

	Little/no progress	Some progress, but stalled	Some progress, and still moving	At my destination!
Not closely following program	Recommit to current program, or change programs.	Recommit to current program *and* add strategies.	Tighten up current program. Add strategies *if* this will not detract from current program.	Exit 14 Maintain
Following program closely	Change behavioral programs. Add cognitive strategies.	Add to current program.	Keep it up! Add strategies only if this will not interfere with current program.	

Thinking about aborting your journey?
Seek help from a behavioral sleep medicine professional!

Figure 13.1. Where to Go From Here

You are at (or close to) your desired destination. It may be tempting to put this book on a shelf and stop working on your sleep. Instead, *turn to chapter 14.* This chapter parallels what we do when we are treating someone with CBT-I: we end with a focus on maintaining progress and decreasing the risk of future insomnia.

You have made progress, and you are still moving in the right direction. If you have made significant progress, your first priority will be to *keep doing what you have been doing.* It is helping, after all! If you have been at all lax in following the strategies you are using, you may want to *recommit and follow your program even more closely* for even better results. For example, if you are sometimes lingering in bed after your alarm goes off, you can tighten up your stimulus control therapy (SCT) or sleep restriction therapy (SRT) program by getting out of bed more quickly. If you have been using designated worry time and have set time aside five days a week, you can increase this to every day.

You may want to *add additional strategies* to your current program. Only do so if this will not interfere with your current program. For example, if you are currently using SCT, you may decide to add SRT for a combined approach. However, if you start to limit your time in bed and find that you are having a harder time getting out of bed when you are not sleeping, then we suggest you go back to using SCT without SRT. Remember, we would rather you use one of these core behavioral treatments fully than two watered-down treatments.

You have made progress, but seem to have stalled out. Again, because you have made some progress, we suggest you *continue to use the strategies you have been using.* However, since you have plateaued short of your goals, we will place a greater emphasis on tweaking your program. Specifically, if you have been closely following your program, then we suggest you *add strategies* to those you already are using.

If you are not fully following the instructions for each strategy you are using, *recommit and follow your program even more closely.* Take some time to reflect. What, specifically, is keeping you from following the program more closely? Is it an issue of willingness? If so, does seeing your partial progress make you more willing to follow the program more closely? Might you benefit from rereading the chapter on willingness? Or are you already willing, but running into practical roadblocks (for example, falling asleep unwittingly before your scheduled bedtime)? Can you do some troubleshooting and get around these blocks?

If you are unwilling to more fully commit, or you simply cannot work around other barriers to your current program, then there are two reasonable options. First is to *add strategies.* This is usually what we would recommend since you are benefiting from what you are doing, even if what you are doing falls short of the "full dose" of the treatment. However, it also is reasonable to *change programs* if you think you will be able to do something else more fully. For example, if you have been using SCT but have a hard time leaving the bed when you wake up in the middle of the night, you may decide that it is time to try SRT.

You have made little or no progress. With little or no progress after six or more weeks, you will want to start something new. However, if you have not been following your program at all closely, then "something new" may mean *recommitting to your current program*! Carefully consider what has gotten in the way. Work to increase willingness and decrease practical roadblocks. Or you may decide to "cut your losses" and *change programs*, rather than put even more time and effort into the program you initially selected, especially if you already have been following your current program closely. If stimulus control has not worked, perhaps sleep restriction will (or vice versa). Or perhaps you can harness the power of both treatments in a combined approach. You also may want to *add strategies* that you are not yet using, such as cognitive strategies or sleep hygiene.

You are out of gas. If you are feeling so stuck or frustrated that you are ready to abandon your journey toward more restorative sleep, then we encourage you to seek the help of a trained professional. It may be time to be evaluated with an overnight sleep study. Or you may benefit from guidance from someone who is practiced in CBT-I.

Common Questions (and Answers) About Planning the Next Leg of Your Adventure

"What do you mean when you suggest that I add strategies?"

Remember that CBT-I is a multicomponent treatment, and there are a lot of tools available. In chapter 5 we helped you pick the strategies that were best suited to your sleep problems, and that you were most willing to do. We suggested you use SCT, SRT, or the combination as your "core" behavioral program. We also suggested that you select one or more cognitive strategies. Now you can add other strategies to what you already are doing.

Think first about which behavioral strategies you are not currently using. Look back at your work in chapter 5 and see if these strategies are safe for you to use. If they are, consider adding one or more. Now think about which cognitive strategies you are not using. Consider adding one or more of these to your toolkit.

Here is a list to help you organize your thoughts. We did not include willingness in this table because it is so integral to every strategy. That is, you are using willingness every time you work your program.

If you are currently using...	You can add...
Stimulus control therapy (SCT)	SRT and/or sleep hygiene
Sleep restriction therapy (SRT)	SCT and/or sleep hygiene
Combined SCT-SRT	Sleep hygiene
Sleep hygiene	SCT and/or SRT
Cognitive restructuring (CR)	DWT, mindfulness, and/or defusion
Designated worry time (DWT)	CR, mindfulness, and/or defusion
Mindfulness	CR, DWT, and/or defusion
Defusion	CR, DWT, and/or mindfulness

"What do you mean when you suggest changing programs?"

Mostly we are referring to changing from one behavioral treatment program to another. Because behavioral strategies have the best research support, we usually do not suggest changing from a behavioral program to a purely cognitive treatment. And since sleep hygiene alone usually does not work, we usually do not suggest that you move to sleep hygiene as your sole behavioral treatment. What's left? You can switch from SCT to SRT, or vice versa. Or you can switch from combined SCT-SRT to either SCT *or* SRT.

You also may choose to change cognitive strategies. For example, maybe you have been using DWT but you realize that you are ruminating (which is the one type of thought process that does not respond well to DWT). You may decide to stop using DWT and use mindfulness and cognitive defusion strategies instead.

"Are all strategies available to me?"

Not necessarily. Be sure to remind yourself whether any of the options you are considering are not suitable (see exercise 5.2).

"Where can I find help if my solo journey is not working for me?"

We suggest you consult with either a physician who is board certified in sleep medicine, or a health provider who specializes in behavioral sleep medicine or CBT for insomnia. Your primary care physician, your insurance company, or a local major medical center may be able to help you locate reputable providers.

Your Next Step

We certainly hope that your sleep, and your relationship with sleep, are better. And we hope these improvements are enough to motivate you to continue on your journey. When you are close to your desired destination, proceed to the next chapter. If you are changing or adding treatment strategies, continue to use a sleep log to track your progress. Read (or reread) relevant chapters so that you are supported in using each treatment strategy correctly. Use willingness and acceptance skills to fully commit to your treatment program and to decrease your struggle with insomnia. Finally, remember to use effectiveness—not rigid rules—as the compass that guides you on the next leg of your journey.

Chapter 14

Maintaining Gains
Across Contexts

Congratulations! You have taken action to improve your sleep. You have read this book. You have created a personalized sleep program. You have implemented this program, and modified it as needed. You have learned what works best for you to promote restorative sleep. Now what? This chapter will help you transition from your sleep program and maintain your gains. We will also address what to do if insomnia starts to creep back into your life. Worksheet 14.1 will help you pull together the work you do in this chapter.

Transitioning from Your Sleep Program

You are likely wondering how long you will need to continue with your personalized sleep program. Is this your new forever? The answer to this question is yes and no. The "yes" answer has to do with your relationship with your sleep. Yes, we want your new perspective about sleep to stay with you. This program has encouraged you to shift from the "fix it now" focus to the "support it over time" focus. We certainly hope this is your new forever. This paradigm shift will allow you to recognize what needs to be done to promote your sleep over your lifetime. This new relationship with sleep will help you quickly recognize when you are pulled into the struggle spiral with sleep. It will help you put down the rope. You will no longer try to control your sleep; as a result, your sleep will have less control over you.

The "no" answer has to do with your day-to-day choices around your sleep. No, you do not have to stick to your personalized sleep program for life. Once you have reliable, restorative sleep, you will naturally consider returning to some of your old habits and patterns, such as reading in bed or sleeping longer when you can. If you are not feeling a strong pull in this direction, then we encourage you to continue with your program. It is working, after all. However, if you do want to make some changes, we have some recommendations.

Decide What to Keep in Place

You probably made at least one change that just feels "right." Even if you resisted it at first, you can tell that this change supports restorative sleep. Going back to your old habit may feel good, in an indulgent kind of way, but you have a strong sense that this would ultimately be unhelpful. Examples from our clients include having a wind-down routine at bedtime, using the bed only for sleep and sex, having a consistent wake time, and using cognitive strategies to quiet their minds.

Based on what we know about sleep physiology, here are our top three recommendations of habits to continue:

Get up within fifteen to thirty minutes of the same time every morning.

Shoot for a somewhat consistent bedtime, but go to bed only when you are sleepy (unless you are never sleepy).

Get out of bed if you are not sleeping and you are getting frustrated or anxious.

Although these are our typical recommendations, everyone is different. You are not "typical." You are you. What aspects of your program do you want to make your way of life? Record your answers on worksheet 14.1.

WORKSHEET 14.1: **Your Sleep Wellness Plan**

Healthy Habits to Continue. These are some of the things I want to continue to do to support restorative sleep and a positive relationship with sleep (for example, maintain a consistent wake time, practice mindfulness):

When to Take Precautions. Things that may *trigger* disrupted sleep in the future include (for example, work stress, relationship stress, travel, physical illness):

Preventive Steps. If any of these triggers are present, I can do these things to make myself less vulnerable to a sleep disruption (for example, have a more regular sleep schedule, decrease caffeine, prioritize my nightly bedtime routine/buffer):

If I have a **LAPSE** (a temporary sleep disruption)...

...I may have these **thoughts** that could start an insomnia spiral:	I want to respond with these **more helpful thoughts**:

197

...I may be tempted to engage in these **compensatory behaviors**:	I can instead choose these **more effective behaviors**:

If I have a **RELAPSE** (longer-term sleep disruption), these are the action steps I will take (for example, stimulus control, decrease struggle/increase acceptance, set designated worry time, make a new treatment plan):

1.

2.

3.

4.

Change One Element at a Time

Some of the behaviors that were helpful as you "worked a program" for insomnia will seem less important to continue. Perhaps you would like to take an occasional nap, sleep in on weekends, and drink more caffeine. Changing several things at once creates more stress for your body than does making one change. It also makes it difficult to assess the effect of each change on your sleep.

Start with the behavior you most want to change. Track your sleep and how you are feeling during the day. After a couple of weeks, take a moment to review the information you have gathered. If your sleep is less restorative, ask yourself if what you gained is worth this setback. Also ask yourself what you think will happen to your sleep if you continue with this particular deviation from your program. If the cost has been great enough, or you see danger ahead, you can return to your program.

If, on the other hand, your sleep is stable after making a move away from your program, then you can take on the next change you want to make. Repeat this process, always tracking the effect so you can make an informed decision about how to best support your sleep moving forward.

Use Your Sleep Log

Most people stop using a sleep log once they are sleeping better. We encourage you to make flexible use of this tool moving forward. You may decide to complete it for one week each month. This will give you a snapshot of your current sleep habits. For example, you will see how consistent versus erratic your sleep-wake schedule is. If it has strayed from the degree of consistency that best supports your sleep, you can quickly self-correct, before you even experience sleep disruption.

You also may want to return to tracking your sleep at the first signs of any sleep disruption, or even when you are facing potential precipitating events. Finally, use a sleep log when you want to see the effect of a change, such as changing medications or your sleep schedule.

Remember to use your sleep log with an attitude of curiosity, not hypervigilance. You are simply collecting data. This data will help you use effectiveness to guide your choices.

Anticipate Triggers for Sleep Disruption

Consider all you have learned about sleep and about your own insomnia spiral. What types of life events are most likely to disrupt your sleep? Work stress? Relationship stress? Being awoken night after night by others (for example, a baby or sick family member)? Physical pain or illness? Record your answers on worksheet 14.1.

One of the most common sleep disruptors is a schedule change. Pay attention. Are the holidays coming up? Do you have travel plans? Is Daylight Savings Time starting or ending? Is your work schedule changing drastically? To maintain your gains, prepare for schedule changes. For example, consider shifting your sleep schedule slowly rather than all at once. Or stay on your normal sleep-wake schedule even when you have time off from work or school.

When trying to determine how you want to handle the situations that put you at risk for sleep disruption, remember the sweet spot. Be watchful, but not hypervigilant. Take proactive steps to keep yourself on track, without being overly controlling and getting into a tug of war.

Responding to Lapses and Relapses

Did we just say do not get into a tug of war? What we meant to say is, notice *when* you get in a tug of war! Then drop the rope, before you get sucked down the insomnia spiral.

We all experience sleep disruption from time to time. A night or two of too little sleep or of poor-quality sleep is to be expected. We call a temporary setback a "lapse." If your brain responds to a lapse by sounding the alarms, or with "quick fix" compensatory behaviors, then a lapse can turn into a "relapse"—a full return of insomnia.

Use worksheet 14.1 to prepare for the lapses you are sure to experience. What types of negative thoughts will your mind likely serve up? Will you jump to the conclusion that insomnia is back and here to stay? Will you struggle rather than accept your experience, telling yourself that you *have* to sleep, *now*? Will you worry about how you will get through tomorrow? Consider how you want to talk back to these negative thoughts. What are more realistic or helpful thoughts? How can you lean into your experience rather than struggle against it?

Now do the same exercise for behaviors. Will you have the urge to spend more time in bed to "make up" for the lost sleep? What would be a more effective choice?

We are optimistic that the knowledge and skills you gained using this workbook will help you ride out brief sleep disruptions without getting caught up in an insomnia spiral. But what if you do experience a relapse?

This is when we encourage you to return to a full CBT-ACT for insomnia program. The quicker the better. It takes less effort to stop a train that is slowly rolling out of the station than to stop a train that has been going full throttle for miles. Similarly, you want to stop the insomnia spiral before it picks up too much speed. Be prepared by knowing what parts of your program you are likely to use, based on your past experience. Go ahead and record this on worksheet 14.1.

If a lot of time has passed, or if your insomnia is of a different flavor, you may want to work through chapter 5 to develop a new plan. All of the worksheets are available electronically if you want fresh copies.

Remember: Sleep to Live, Don't Live to Sleep

We also can think of lapses and relapses in terms of your behaviors, rather than of your sleep itself. That is, you can revert back to sleep-interfering behaviors but then quickly correct (a lapse), or you can get sucked into old patterns for weeks or months (a relapse).

Lapses are the unavoidable result of living your life fully. As odd as this may sound, they are the key to your continued success. These natural fluctuations are a sign of flexibility. And this flexibility is necessary for a long-term sustainable relationship with sleep.

For example, if you spend the weekend with some friends you may choose to stay up late each night and sleep in each morning. You may even take a nap. If you return to your usual schedule Monday morning, then you had a brief lapse into potentially sleep-interfering behaviors. And this lapse was in the service of spending meaningful time with friends. You let sleep support living.

But you also let sleep support living by quickly getting back to a more consistent schedule. This promotes restorative sleep over the long term, which promotes a better quality of life. Now imagine that your one weekend of flexibility turns into weeks of an erratic sleep schedule. Your behavioral lapse has turned into a relapse. This is more risky. There is a greater chance that you will lose gains in your sleep. Ironically, the more poorly you are sleeping, the more you will start to revolve your life around sleep.

We are back to the idea of the sweet spot. We encourage you to be flexible enough to support a rich and vital life, but not so flexible that you are undermining your body's natural ability to sleep.

Your Next Step

Anything you care about requires some nurturing. Sleep is no exception. Continue to promote restorative sleep throughout your life. Keep doing the things that support your body's natural ability to sleep. Be aware of what may disrupt your sleep, and take precautions when these potential triggers are present. When you first experience sleep disruption, respond, but do not overrespond. If insomnia returns in full force, return to your CBT-ACT program. And, through it all, try to be willing to have whatever this particular night brings.

Chapter 15

Last Words

This book is about our knowledge and your wisdom. Our knowledge is based on science, research, and clinical practice. Your wisdom is based on your personal and unique set of strengths, challenges, and circumstances. You know yourself better than anyone else. Integrating our knowledge and your wisdom leads to an optimal sleep program.

The most effective intervention for insomnia today is CBT-I. This program helps you get unstuck by addressing the thoughts and behaviors that feed your insomnia spiral. Unfortunately, it can be challenging to follow this program. CBT-I requires short-term discomfort, a willingness to change, and patience and trust in the process. We use ACT strategies to help you more fully embrace CBT-I.

Our hybrid CBT-ACT for insomnia program addresses three challenges inherent in CBT-I as it is typically delivered in self-help books and by sleep doctors and therapists. The first challenge is a one-size-fits-all approach to treating insomnia with CBT-I. We address this by personalizing CBT-I to your unique needs. The second challenge is that CBT-I is often delivered in an overly rigid fashion. The people receiving CBT-I may take on this rigid approach, or may not follow the program closely enough. We address this by encouraging willingness and flexibility, both in creating and in executing your program. We also address this by using effectiveness, rather than rigid rules, to guide your treatment. The third challenge is the assumption that CBT-I can be used to control your sleep. We address this by debunking this myth. For people struggling with insomnia, control is a problem, not a solution.

Here are the key take-home messages that we hope we conveyed to you:

- Your brain knows how to sleep. You just have to get out of its way.

- Your relationship with sleep matters. You cannot control sleep. If you try, it will control you. Take the time to develop a sustainable relationship that focuses on long-term health rather than short-term fixes. This is the paradigm shift.

- Struggling with insomnia (or your sleep program) does not promote restorative sleep. Willingness is your countermove.

- Find your sweet spot. CBT-I works—if you really do it. But you do not want to do it so rigidly that it fuels anxiety.

- Your relationship with CBT-I matters. Take the time to develop a personalized program that fits you and your sleep challenges.

- ACT supports a flexible relationship with both sleep and CBT-I. Willingness, mindfulness, and cognitive defusion strategies facilitate sleep-promoting thoughts and behaviors.

- Effectiveness—what works in the long term—is the best compass to guide your sleep-related choices.

- Sleep to live, do not live to sleep!

Thank you for allowing us to accompany you on your journey. We hope that our hybrid CBT-ACT program has helped you end your insomnia struggle, restoring both your sleep and your relationship with sleep.

Acknowledgments

We are indebted to Ruth Rotkowitz, Dr. Vyga Kaufmann, Dr. Natalie Whiteford, and Susan Brosse for reading earlier drafts of this workbook. Your constructive feedback greatly improved the final product, and your encouragement helped sustain us on our writing journey. We thank Dr. Michael Weissberg, who was the first to urge us to apply our skills as cognitive behavioral therapists to the treatment of insomnia. We additionally thank him and all of the other doctors and therapists who have entrusted their patients to us. We are so appreciative of the people who have sought our help when feeling sleep deprived and vulnerable. It was you who taught us the importance of blending cognitive behavior therapy and acceptance and commitment therapy for better results. Thank you for letting us help you find your "sweet spot." It has been extremely rewarding to treat so many people with insomnia, given the high success rate and relatively quick results. A heartfelt thank you to everyone at New Harbinger Publications who contributed to the production of this workbook. Finally, we thank our families who endured us working on beach vacations and over the Thanksgiving holiday to complete this project. Your understanding and support are immensely appreciated.

Circadian Rhythm Disorders

Circadian rhythm disorders affect the *timing* of your sleep. When you have a circadian rhythm disorder, your body clock is not in alignment with the world's clock. Your body is able to sleep but not at the times you want or need to. There are two explanations for these types of sleep problems. One explanation is that your body clock is not working properly. Disorders resulting from a dysfunctional body clock include delayed sleep phase syndrome, advanced sleep phase syndrome, irregular sleep-wake rhythm disorder, and free-running disorder.

The other explanation for circadian rhythm disorders is that your work and social obligations are misaligned with the external clock. Disorders resulting from this misalignment include jet lag and shift-work disorder.

We are going to focus specifically on advanced and delayed sleep phase syndromes in this chapter. These are the two most common circadian rhythm disorders to be confused with insomnia.

Do You Have a Sleep Preference or a Sleep Problem?

There is variation in when people are primed for sleep. None of these variations are problematic in and of themselves. If you can accommodate your body's schedule and get restorative sleep, we consider your shifted schedule to be a preference, not a problem.

Problems arise when your body's natural sleep window does not mesh with your life. For example, you may be sleep deprived because you have to be up and about when your body is primed to sleep, and you can only sleep for part of the time you have set aside for sleep.

Or you may be sacrificing important parts of your life (for example, job opportunities or social engagements) to accommodate your body clock. If your shifted body clock is causing this kind of distress or discomfort, then we call it a circadian rhythm disorder.

If you prefer to go to bed early and get up early, we call you a *morning lark*. Elderly people are most likely to have this sleep schedule. As long as you enjoy this schedule *and* it supports your daily obligations, this is not a problem. It is your body's preference. However, if this pattern is interfering with your life or causing sleep deprivation, you may have a circadian rhythm disorder known as *advanced sleep phase syndrome*. The name comes from the current timing of your sleep opportunity. The time during which you are able to sleep is advanced, or ahead of, what you would like it, or need it, to be.

Advanced sleep phase syndrome can look like insomnia of the early awakening type. You may push through the early hours of your body's sleep opportunity to be on a "normal" schedule. When you finally climb into bed you fall asleep easily because your body is primed to sleep. However, your wake drive then pulls you out of sleep before you have gotten enough hours. To your body clock, the next day has begun.

If you prefer to go to bed late and get up late, we call you a *night owl*. Adolescents and young adults are most likely to have this sleep schedule. As long as you enjoy this schedule *and* it supports your daily obligations, this is not a problem. It is your body's preference. However, if this pattern is interfering with your life or causing sleep deprivation, you may have a circadian rhythm disorder known as *delayed sleep phase syndrome*. The name comes from the current timing of your sleep opportunity. The time during which you are able to sleep is delayed, or behind, what you would like it, or need it, to be.

Delayed sleep phase syndrome can look like the type of insomnia marked by trouble falling asleep. If you have to wake up earlier than your body clock would prefer, it is natural to also try to go to sleep earlier, so that you can get the hours you need. Unfortunately, your body is not yet primed for sleep, so you lie awake until it is.

Accommodating Your Body's Natural Rhythm

One way to treat advanced and delayed sleep phase syndromes is to arrange your life around your body's natural schedule. Remember, a body clock that is out of sync with the external clock is not unhealthy or dangerous in any way. It is only a problem when it interferes with your life. If you are able to stop fighting it, this is a perfectly reasonable treatment!

What would you have to do to accommodate your natural rhythm? For example, would you have to request different work hours, or start to work for yourself instead of for others? Would you have to negotiate different responsibilities at home? Would you have to change what you do in your leisure time, because different social opportunities are available? Would you see certain people you care about less?

Now consider what you would stand to gain if you accepted your circadian rhythm as it is. Would it be a relief to stop fighting it? Would you get more restorative sleep? Could your sleep schedule complement your partner's, or your coworkers'?

If you think you would gain more than you would sacrifice, you may want to try this approach to dealing with your body clock's misalignment with the external clock. But what if accommodating your body clock would come at too great a cost?

Shifting Your Body's Schedule

Multiple strategies can help you shift the timing of your sleep schedule. These include behavioral therapy, light therapy, melatonin, and chronotherapy.

Behavioral Therapy

We use the components of CBT-I in a slightly different way when trying to shift your clock. The behavioral components of CBT-I are used not only to promote restorative sleep, but also to move the sleep cycle to a different time. Therefore you will be focusing not just on what behaviors you engage in to promote your sleep cycle, but also on when you are going to engage in these behaviors.

MOVING YOUR BEDTIME AND WAKE TIME

If you have advanced sleep phase syndrome, you will want to move your bedtime later in the evening and your wake time later in the morning. It will be easier for you to manipulate the time you go to bed: you can force yourself to stay up for an additional fifteen minutes, but you cannot force your body to sleep fifteen minutes later.

If you have delayed sleep phase syndrome, you will want to move your bedtime earlier in the night and your wake time earlier in the morning. It will be easier for you to manipulate the time you wake up: you can force yourself to get up earlier, but you cannot force yourself to fall asleep earlier.

Put your primary focus on the part of your sleep schedule that you have more control over. The other will hopefully follow. It is recommended that you shift your bedtime and wake time in increments of fifteen minutes every three to five days. We do not recommend that you make a drastic shift in your bedtime or wake time. Our bodies are built for gradual change.

For example, let's say you have been going to bed at 2 a.m. and waking at 9 a.m. (for a total of seven hours' time in bed), but want to sleep eight hours a night, going to bed at 10 p.m. and waking at 6 a.m. The first step is to set your alarm and wake at 8:45 a.m. You will have a target bedtime of 1:45 a.m. Use this schedule for three to five days. Then start to wake up at 8:30 a.m. and climb into bed at 1:30 a.m. Repeat this schedule for three to five days. Continue to shift in fifteen-minute increments until you reach your desired goal of 10 p.m. to 6 a.m.

DELIBERATE TIMING OF YOUR ACTIVITIES

Be mindful of *when* you do activities that are engaging. If you have advanced sleep phase syndrome, you will want to add engaging activities in the late afternoon and evening and remove them from the early morning hours. If you have delayed sleep phase syndrome, you will want to decrease engaging activities in the evening and add them to your mornings. This sounds easier than it is. There are lots of activities that are more activating than we initially realize. Return to the section "Stimulus Control Therapy: Detailed Instructions" in chapter 6 for a full review on how to replace activating activities with more calming options.

ROUTINE AS AN ANCHOR

It is very important to routinize your schedule as much as possible. Whenever possible, exercise at the same time every day. If you can, time your exercise to occur at approximately four to five hours before your desired bedtime. If this is not possible, then add in an activity that will create core heat in your body approximately four to five hours before your desired bedtime. Climbing stairs or doing jumping jacks are examples. As little as five minutes is all you need to create a little heat in your body. This heat is in sync with the sleep cycle you are promoting.

Eat at least one meal at the same time every day. Consistent digestion will help you anchor the sleep cycle you are promoting.

SLEEP HYGIENE

Using sleep hygiene can be very effective to shift your sleep schedule. The goal is to provide your body with as many cues as you can to sleep at the time you want to be sleeping. Refer to chapter 9 for a full review of sleep hygiene.

Light Therapy

Circadian rhythm disorders are also treated with light therapy. You may remember from chapter 2 that light is one of the main influences on sleep from our external world. Light cues your mind and body to be awake. Darkness cues your mind and body to sleep. Light therapy involves adding and blocking light at strategic times to encourage your body to shift its sleep-wake cycles. Light therapy is one of the most effective tools in shifting the time of your sleep cycle.

ADVANCED SLEEP PHASE SYNDROME

Your body is currently wired to fall asleep before your desired bedtime. What cues your body to be awake? Light. Therefore, it is important to provide light in the late afternoon hours. Get outside or use a light that mimics daylight between 3 p.m. and 6 p.m. This light will cue your body clock to stay awake for a longer period of time. After repeated exposure to light at this time, your body clock will shift the timing of your sleep to a later point.

You are also wired to wake up before your desired wake time. What cues your body to stay asleep? Darkness. Therefore, it is important to block light in the early morning hours. Remain in a dark or semidark environment until 5 a.m. This environment will send a cue to your body clock to stay asleep later. After repeated exposure to darkness at this time, your body clock will shift the timing of your awakening to a later point.

DELAYED SLEEP PHASE SYNDROME

Your body is currently wired to fall asleep after your desired bedtime. What cues your body to fall asleep? Darkness. Therefore, it is important to increase darkness in the evening hours. You will want to (partially) block light between 6 p.m. and 9 p.m. This environment sends a cue to your body clock to initiate sleep. After repeated exposure to darkness at this time, your body clock will shift the timing of your sleep to an earlier point.

You are also wired to wake up later than your desired wake time. What cues your body to be awake? Light. Therefore, it is important to provide light in the morning hours. Throw open the curtains, get outside, or use a light that mimics daylight within the first hour of your desired wake time. This light sends the cue to your body clock to start your wake cycle. After repeated exposure to light at this time, your body clock will shift the timing of your awakening to an earlier point.

ADDING LIGHT

Not all lights are the same. The best light source is natural light. If you live in an environment that has ample sunshine, then you can use this invaluable resource. You can benefit from natural light by going outside or by sitting inside near a window. You do not need to face the sun or stare directly at the sun. You just need to be exposed to the light.

If you do not have access to natural light at the appropriate times, there are many options for artificial light. You want to look for bulbs or lamps that mimic natural light. This means an intensity of around 2500 lux. Recent studies indicate that using a light source below 2500 lux is not effective for shifting your sleep cycle (Dewan et al., 2011). These light sources are not expensive (around $40) and are readily available.

You may be tempted to buy a higher lux light. After all, bigger is better, right? This is not necessarily the case with this intervention. If you are exposed to too much light (5000–10,000 lux), it can have a reverse effect. Too much light can cause irritability, anxiety, and trouble sleeping. Therefore, we highly recommend that you start with the lower levels first. Track your progress before you increase the brightness of your light.

There are specific cases in which you do *not* want to use higher levels of light for your sleep. If you have bipolar disorder or a family history of bipolar disorder, please be very careful using light therapy. Too much light can trigger a manic episode. If you have any current problems with your eyes or are taking photosensitizing medications, you will want to avoid light therapy. About a third of migraine sufferers have adverse effects with light therapy. Having a seizure disorder is another contraindication. If you have *any* concerns, we strongly encourage you talk to your medical providers before using light for your sleep.

These same parameters hold true for determining the duration of your light exposure. More is not necessarily better. Historically, it was thought that a shorter exposure of high-intensity light was most effective. More recently, studies have shown that a longer period of moderate-intensity light may be more effective for circadian rhythm disorders (Dewan et al., 2011).

BLOCKING LIGHT

Prior to the invention of electricity, we had much lower levels of sleep disorders. Electricity is a wonderful addition to our daily lives, but can be an impediment to our sleep.

There are many accessible and cost-effective ways to block light. The most effective method is to turn off your lights. There is no confusion when it is dark. Your body knows this means it is time to sleep. You can put light-blocking curtains (or dark sheets or blankets) over your windows as needed. You can use an eye mask as needed.

Of course, you will not be asleep the entire time that you want to be in relative darkness. This means you will need some light even during these times. Choose low light as much as possible. You can install dimmer switches on your lights to turn them down. You can use lamps with twenty-five-watt bulbs instead of overhead lights.

Also choose lights that do not contain blue light. Blue spectrum light most closely mimics daylight. Human brains evolved with fire as the only source of light after sundown, and fire does not contain the blue wavelength of light. Blue light is found in standard, compact fluorescent, and LED light bulbs, flat-screen televisions, smartphones and tablets, and most computer screens.

Whenever possible we suggest you not use electronic devices when you are trying to be in darkness. Again, removing the light completely is the most optimal treatment. If this is not possible, there are alternatives. There are apps you can download to your devices that block the blue light. You can purchase orange gels that cover your devices, again blocking the blue light. You also can purchase sunglasses that are designed to block the blue wavelength of light. This is the most versatile option, as you can move from one device or room to another, with continuous protection from blue light.

Melatonin

Melatonin is a popular supplement for sleep. It is readily available and affordable. Most people use melatonin as a hypnotic. They take it at bedtime since melatonin can make you sleepy at higher doses. However, melatonin also can be used to advance your body clock if you take it early enough. Taking microdoses (0.3 to 0.5 mg) of melatonin several hours before the desired bedtime can help you shift your schedule earlier if you have delayed sleep phase syndrome.

However, we suggest that you proceed with caution if you decide to use melatonin. Melatonin, like any substance you ingest, comes with both benefits and risks. Melatonin is not regulated by the FDA, so quality and dosage are not monitored. Melatonin can interact with other medications and supplements you are taking. Not all people benefit from using melatonin. We encourage you to consult with your medical providers prior to using melatonin or other supplements.

Chronotherapy

Chronotherapy is a very specific treatment for delayed sleep phase syndrome. You may already be aware that it is easier to keep yourself awake when you are sleepy than it is to go to bed when you are not. As a result, it is often quite challenging for people to gradually shift their sleep schedule forward in the manner we suggested earlier. Chronotherapy takes a backdoor approach to manage this barrier. Instead of trying to move the sleep cycle forward, you move it backwards (later). You keep moving the cycle backwards until you have gone all the way around the clock! When your sleep cycle reaches the desired time point, you maintain the new sleep schedule.

This intervention is extremely challenging. During chronotherapy, there will be times when you are sleeping in the middle of the day and staying awake all night. This takes quite a bit of planning and strategizing. Chronotherapy should be done under the supervision of a sleep specialist. You deserve to have a knowledgeable clinician on your team if you are going to engage in this challenging treatment.

Summary

It is very important to know whether you are treating insomnia or a circadian rhythm disorder. Even the most carefully crafted, well thought-out insomnia program will not be effective if you are treating the wrong thing!

If you do have a circadian rhythm disorder, you may decide to accommodate your body's natural rhythm. Or you may try to shift it. We hope that the tools in this chapter put you on the right track. However, if you are trying to shift your clock by many hours, then we strongly encourage you to work with a sleep specialist. This is a difficult condition to treat, and you will benefit from expert guidance.

Insomnia and Menopause

*M*any of the older women who come to see us say that their insomnia started during perimenopause. Do you remember the 3P model of insomnia from chapter 3? In some ways, perimenopause is no different than any of the other myriad experiences that we can classify as "What Life Gave You." Just like any other change or event, perimenopause interacts with your particular risk factors for sleep disruption. And your response to an initial sleep disruption—what you do and how you think about sleep— will determine whether you get caught up in an insomnia spiral.

Still, there is something unique about the link between menopause and sleep. Unlike other life events, menopause involves specific physiological changes. And there is one menopausal symptom in particular that has been linked to insomnia: hot flashes. Hot flashes are sudden feelings of heat in your upper body (face, neck, chest). You may sweat profusely as your body tries to cool itself down, and then you may feel chilled. It is no wonder, then, that nighttime hot flashes disrupt sleep!

If your insomnia started during perimenopause but you did not experience hot flashes, then there is a good chance that aging, rather than menopause, is to blame. Research suggests that we experience more middle-of-the-night awakenings as we age, and this is independent of menopausal status (Eichling & Sahni, 2005). For example, a forty-three-year-old woman who is postmenopause is less likely to report insomnia than a forty-eight-year-old woman who is premenopause.

What does this mean for you? If you have insomnia that started during perimenopause but you did not experience nighttime hot flashes, then you can use the treatment in this workbook without modification. You also do not need to modify this treatment if hot flashes used to disrupt your sleep but no longer do. We expect our combined CBT-ACT approach to work just as well for you as for someone whose insomnia did not start during perimenopause. Remember: what initially triggered your insomnia may be very different than what is keeping it around. And it is the perpetuating factors, not the initial cause, that we need to target in treatment. This is true even if the cause is menopause or aging.

But maybe you do wake up in a sweat, feeling as if a surge of adrenaline is going through your body. What then? You can treat your hot flashes or you can treat your sleep disturbance—or you can treat them both.

Treat Your Hot Flashes

Remember, research suggests that it is specifically the phenomenon of hot flashes that links menopause and sleep. Therefore, reducing or eliminating your hot flashes should lead to better sleep. For example, in their review of research on menopause-related sleep disorders, Eichling and Sahni (2005) demonstrate that estrogen replacement therapy reduces hot flashes and improves sleep for women who experience hot flashes.

There are a number of treatment options available for hot flashes, including various forms of hormone replacement therapy, acupuncture, and herbal remedies. A thorough discussion of this topic is beyond the scope of this book. Two popular resources that review these options are *The Wisdom of Menopause* (Northrup, 2012) and *The Menopause Book* (Wingert & Kantrowitz, 2009). We encourage you to talk with your physician if nighttime hot flashes are significantly disrupting your sleep.

Treat Your Sleep Disturbance

All of the CBT and ACT strategies discussed in this book can be helpful even if hot flashes are what rudely awaken you from sleep. However, we tend to gravitate toward certain strategies when we are helping women in this situation.

Stimulus Control Therapy (SCT)

SCT gives you a specific plan that you can execute when you wake up in the middle of the night. By leaving your bed, you are less likely to start to mentally link your bed with the feelings of adrenaline and heat. Leaving your bed also may help you cool off more quickly.

Use the same guidelines outlined in chapter 6 to develop your SCT plan. Think about what might be different in light of your hot flashes. For example, should one of the preparations you make ahead of time be having a change of clothes at the ready? Do you want to have two plans for what to do when you leave your room—one for awakenings triggered by hot flashes and one for other awakenings? Perhaps your standard plan will be to go to the den and read, but you expect to be too uncomfortable to do this if you have just had a hot flash. In that case, perhaps you first will take some steps to help you cool off (or to warm up if you are chilled).

Why do we generally suggest SCT over sleep restriction therapy (SRT) when hot flashes are involved? In SRT we are trying to prevent awakenings by consolidating your sleep. It is not realistic to think that you will sleep through a hot flash no matter how deeply you are sleeping! Also, your experience of night sweats may be pretty erratic. This means that your average sleep efficiency may be over 90%, even though you have some nights with long awakenings. This pattern guides us to SCT over SRT.

Hot Flash–Specific Sleep Hygiene

You may need a different sleep environment when you are prone to hot flashes. To what temperature is your thermostat set at night? Is there a different setting that would be more comfortable right now? Consider layers of bedding instead of one warm comforter, so you can adjust to your body's shifting needs. Some women swear by "cooling pillows" to help stave off night sweats.

Your hot flashes also may be related to other sleep hygiene guidelines. Consider adding hot flashes to your sleep log to see if you can see any patterns. For example, too much caffeine can increase hot flashes. Spicy food can, too. Finally, many women report that stress brings on their hot flashes. Consider a relaxing wind-down routine to help you reduce stress at bedtime.

Acceptance-Based Strategies

Willingness can help you relate differently not only to your sleep, but also to the hot flashes themselves. Struggling against your experience—wanting the hot flashes to *stop!*—does not help. You can cultivate self-compassion by acknowledging that you are extremely uncomfortable. You can, simultaneously, accept that this is part of your experience as your body transitions into menopause. Your willingness to experience this particular hot flash, on this particular night—and the sleep disruption that comes with it—will keep you from feeding the insomnia spiral.

Some women find mindfulness meditation exercises helpful in calming their nervous system in the aftermath of a hot flash. Consider practicing mindfulness if you leave your bed as part of SCT. You also may want to seek out mindfulness exercises that are specifically focused on cultivating self-compassion. Your body is experiencing significant changes and it can be a wild ride! Treating yourself kindly can help buffer you from stressful aspects of the menopausal transition.

Your Next Step

If you experience nighttime hot flashes that disrupt your sleep, first ask yourself if sleep disruption has taken on a life of its own. Do you have trouble falling or staying asleep that is not directly related to a hot flash? If so, use this workbook to treat your insomnia. Consider the menopause-specific tips in this chapter when you develop your personalized sleep program. Also consider consulting a health professional about strategies for reducing hot flashes.

If your sleep disruption has *not* taken on a life of its own, consider using this workbook to keep it from doing so. Part 1 should be especially useful. This is where you might focus your attention:

Educate yourself about the insomnia spiral (chapter 3), so you can avoid common pitfalls in your response to your sleep disruption.

Use effectiveness as your guide (chapter 1). If your body is craving more sleep as it navigates all the hormonal changes of menopause, try giving it what it is asking for. If you sleep and feel better, continue to listen to your body. If, on the other hand, your sleep simply thins out to cover the wider territory you have set aside for it, then staying in bed longer is an unhelpful compensatory strategy that will feed insomnia.

Practice acceptance and willingness (chapter 4). Try to find your sweet spot: can you be proactive in trying to minimize your physical discomfort, without struggling to control your hot flashes or your sleep?

Like so many other life events and transitions, menopause can make you vulnerable to sleep disruption. How you respond can make all the difference. Understanding and making use of CBT and ACT principles can help you avoid, or get untangled from, the insomnia spiral.

References

Ansfield, M., D. Wegner, and R. Bowser. 1996. "Ironic Effects of Sleep Urgency." *Behavioral Research Therapy* 34: 523–531.

Bootzin, R., and M. Perlis. 2011. "Stimulus Control Therapy." In *Behavioral Treatments for Sleep Disorders: A Comprehensive Primer of Behavioral Sleep Medicine Interventions*, edited by M. Perlis, M. Aloia, and B. Kuhn. London: Academic Press.

Borbely, A. 1982. "A Two Process Model of Sleep Regulation." *Human Neurobiology* 1: 195–204.

Dewan, K., S. Benloucif, K. Reid, L. Wolfe, and P. Zee. 2011. "Light-Induced Changes of the Circadian Clock of Humans: Increasing Duration Is More Effective Than Increasing Light Intensity." *Sleep* 34: 593–599.

Eichling, P., and J. Sahni. 2005. "Menopause Related Sleep Disorders." *Journal of Clinical Sleep Medicine* 1: 291–300.

Espie, C., N. Broomfield, K. MacMahon, L. Macphee, and L. Taylor. 2006. "The Attention-Intention-Effort Pathway in the Development of Psychophysiological Insomnia: A Theoretical Review." *Sleep Medicine Review* 10: 215–245.

Glovinsky, P., and A. Spielman. 2006. *The Insomnia Answer*. New York: Perigee.

Halberg, F. 1969. "Chronobiology." *Annual Review of Physiology* 31: 675–725.

Harvey, A. 2001. "A Cognitive Model of Insomnia." *Behaviour Research and Therapy* 40: 869–893.

Harvey, A., L. Bélanger, L. Talbot, P. Eidelman, S. Beaulieu-Bonneau, E. Fortier-Brochu, et al. 2014. "Comparative Efficacy of Behavior Therapy, Cognitive Therapy, and Cognitive Behavior Therapy for Chronic Insomnia: A Randomized Controlled Trial." *Journal of Consulting and Clinical Psychology* 82: 670–683.

Hölzel, B., J. Carmody, M. Vangel, C. Congleton, S. Yerramsetti, T. Gard, and S. Lazar. 2011. "Mindfulness Practice Leads to Increases in Regional Brain Gray Matter Density." *Psychiatry Research* 191: 36–43.

Jefferson, C., C. Drake, H. Scofield, E. Myers, T. McClure, T. Roehrs, and T. Roth. 2005. "Sleep Hygiene Practices in a Population-Based Sample of Insomniacs." *Sleep* 28: 611–615.

Lundh, L.-G., and H. Hindmarsh. 2002. "Can Meta-cognitive Observation Be Used in the Treatment of Insomnia? A Pilot Study of a Cognitive-Emotional Self-Observation Task." *Behavioural and Cognitive Psychotherapy* 30: 233–236.

Manber, R., R. Bootzin, C. Acebo, and M. Carskadon. 1996. "The Effects of Regularizing Sleep-Wake Schedules on Daytime Sleepiness." *Sleep* 19: 432–441.

McGowan, S., and E. Behar. 2013. "A Preliminary Investigation of Stimulus Control Training for Worry: Effects on Anxiety and Insomnia." *Behavior Modification* 37: 90–112

Mitchell, M., P. Gehrman, M. Perlis, and C. Umscheid. 2012. "Comparative Effectiveness of Cognitive Behavioral Therapy for Insomnia: A Systematic Review." *BMC Family Practice* 13: 40.

Morin, C., R. Bootzin, D. Buysse, J. Edinger, C. Espie, and K. Lichstein. 2006. "Psychological and Behavioral Treatment of Insomnia: Update of the Recent Evidence (1998–2004)." *Sleep* 29: 1398–1414.

National Institutes of Health. 2005. "National Institutes of Health State of the Science Conference Statement on Manifestations and Management of Chronic Insomnia in Adults." *Sleep* 28: 1049–1057.

Nofzinger, E., D. Buysse, A. Germain, J. Price, J. Miewald, and D. Kupfer. 2004. "Functional Neuroimaging Evidence for Hyperarousal in Insomnia." *American Journal of Psychiatry* 161: 2126–2128.

Northrup, C. 2012. *The Wisdom of Menopause: Creating Physical and Emotional Health During the Change.* New York: Bantam.

Ong, J., and D. Sholtes. 2010. "A Mindfulness-Based Approach to the Treatment of Insomnia." *Journal of Clinical Psychology* 66: 1175–1184.

Smith, L., S. Nowakowski, J. Soeffing, H. Orff, and M. Perlis. 2003. "The Measurement of Sleep." In *Treating Sleep Disorders: Principles and Practices of Behavioral Sleep Medicine*, edited by M. Perlis and K. Lichstein. New Jersey: Wiley.

Spielman, A., Y. Chien-Ming, and P. Glovinsky. 2011. "Sleep Restriction Therapy." In *Behavioral Treatment for Sleep Disorders: A Comprehensive Primer of Behavioral Sleep Medicine Interventions*, edited by M. Perlis, M. Aloia, and B. Kuhn. London: Academic Press.

Wever, R. 1979. *The Circadian System of Man: Results of Experiments Under Temporal Isolation.* New York: Springer Verlag.

Williams, R., I. Karacan, and C. Hursch. 1974. *EEG of Human Sleep: Clinical Applications.* New York: Wiley.

Wingert, P., and B. Kantrowitz. 2009. *The Menopause Book.* New York: Workman Publishing.

Colleen Ehrnstrom, PhD, ABPP, is a licensed clinical psychologist who specializes in acceptance and commitment therapy (ACT). She is board certified in cognitive behavioral therapy (CBT), and works in the family program at the Department of Veterans Affairs in Denver, CO.

Alisha L. Brosse, PhD, is a licensed clinical psychologist who specializes in behavioral therapies for a wide range of presenting problems, especially sleep, mood, and anxiety disorders. She operates a private practice in Boulder, CO, and directs a bipolar specialty clinic at the University of Colorado Boulder.

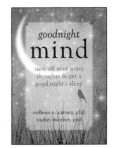
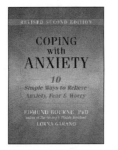
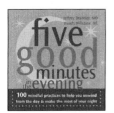
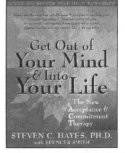
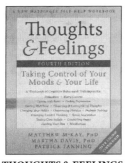
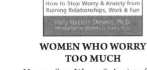
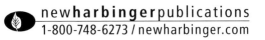

Register your **new harbinger** titles for additional benefits!

When you register your **new harbinger** title—purchased in any format, from any source—you get access to benefits like the following:

- Downloadable accessories like printable worksheets and extra content

- Instructional videos and audio files

- Information about updates, corrections, and new editions

Not every title has accessories, but we're adding new material all the time.

Access free accessories in 3 easy steps:

1. Sign in at NewHarbinger.com (or **register** to create an account).

2. Click on **register a book**. Search for your title and click the **register** button when it appears.

3. Click on the **book cover or title** to go to its details page. Click on **accessories** to view and access files.

That's all there is to it!

If you need help, visit:

NewHarbinger.com/accessories

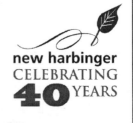

new harbinger
CELEBRATING
40 YEARS